Praise for *Fewer Pills, More Paws*

"*Fewer Pills, More Paws* offers a thoughtful and creatively woven exploration of neuroscience, pharmacology, and insights drawn from our relationships with pets, all in the context of supporting individuals in the aging journey. It encourages readers to pause and consider alternative approaches that may be equally effective before automatically defaulting to medication in some situations. It provides explanations of brain processes that are clear and accessible, making complex concepts easy to grasp. The author also provides practical strategies and mindset shifts that may help ease challenges for all involved. This is an interesting and engaging read."

— **Teepa Snow**
Founder of Positive Approach to Care®

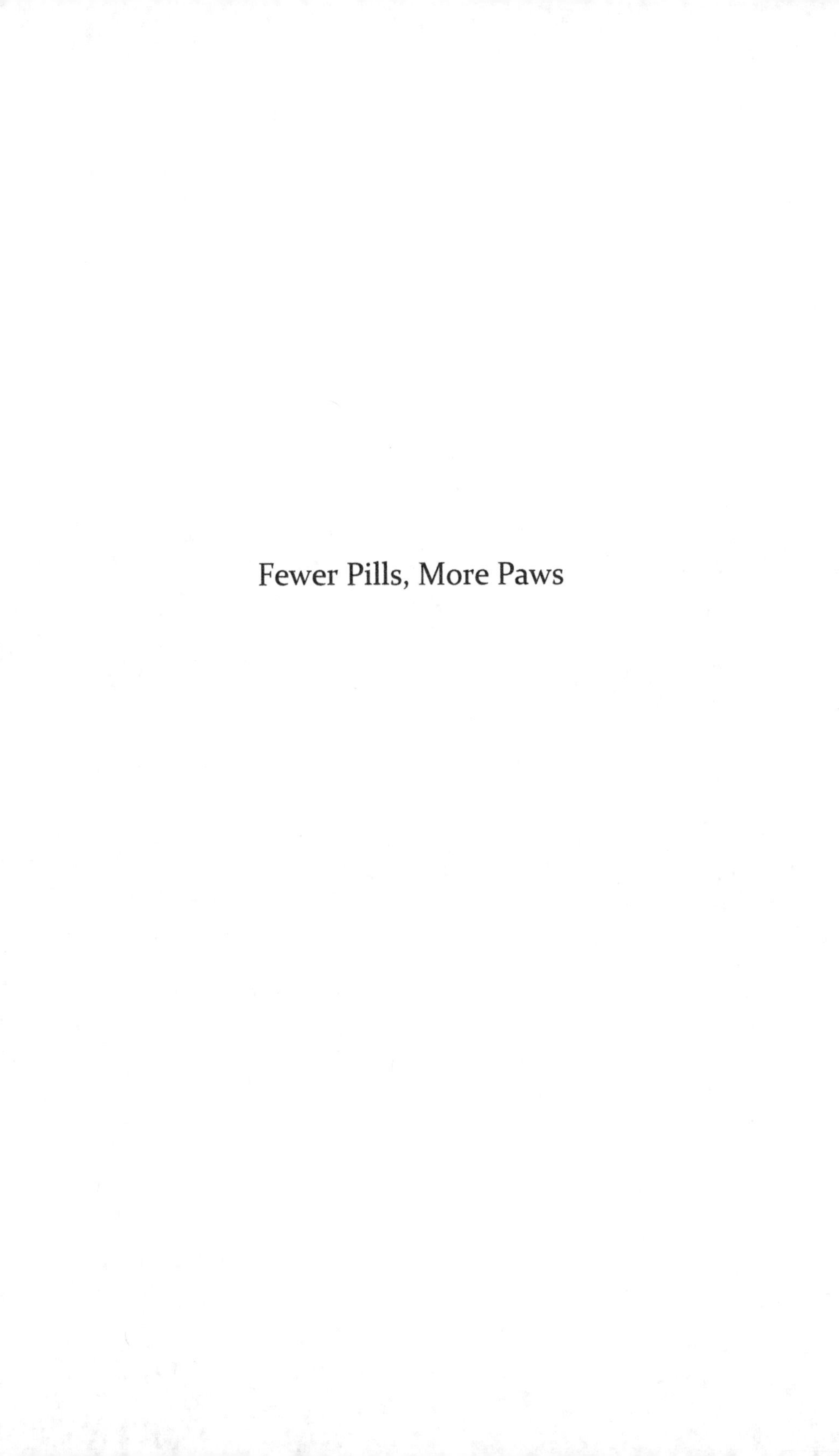

Fewer Pills, More Paws

Fewer Pills, More Paws

Caring for Your Aging Parents and Lessons from Our Pets

David Lee, PharmD, PhD
Founder of MyRxPro

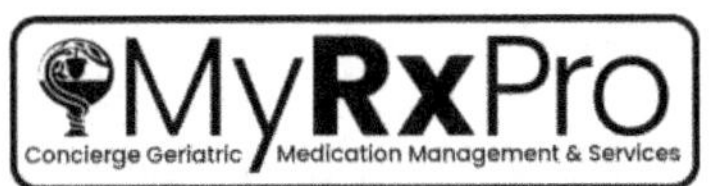

MyRxPro Press
PO Box 80296, Portland, Oregon 97280
MyRxPro.com

Edited by Monica Franz
Cover Design: Anastasia Gilliam
Cover Layout: Max Tower

Printed in The United States.

ISBN: 979-8-9944589-0-7 (eBook)
ISBN: 979-8-9944589-1-4 (Paperback)
ISBN: 979-8-9944589-3-8 (Audiobook - Retail)
ISBN: 979-8-9944589-4-5 (Audiobook - Library)
ISBN: 979-8-9944589-5-2 (Hardcover)

First Edition

Dedication

To Jürgen Venitz, my mentor & the teacher I strive to be.

Table of Contents

I am tired.

Not the tired that sleep fixes. The tired that comes from watching the same preventable harm happen over and over again—in hospitals, in nursing homes, in the bedrooms of families who trusted the system to help their aging parent and watched, instead, as that parent became someone they didn't recognize.

I am a pharmacist. I have spent years watching seniors prescribed 15, sometimes 20 different medications. High-potency medications. Medications that interact with each other in ways that no one is tracking. Medications that accumulate in aging kidneys and aging livers, building up to toxic levels. The brain is brewing in a chemical fog. A dozen medications that were never meant to be used together, but are—because no one is paying attention to the whole picture.

It's like watching a tightrope walker in a hurricane. The human body is resilient—astonishingly resilient—but at some point, the forces working against it become too great. It's a testament to the strength of aging bodies that they stay upright on that tightrope as long as they do.

But here's what breaks my heart: it doesn't have to be this way.

I watch antipsychotics prescribed off-label, day after day, in every hospital I walk through. The evidence against this practice is clear, peer-reviewed, unambiguous. It has been for decades. It's dangerous. It's reckless. And it happens constantly. I see those patients go home sedated, confused, diminished. I watch their families try to get them back—switching medications, adjusting doses, hoping something will work. Some of them recover. Many don't.

They are gone, while their bodies just keep going.

I see families struggle with simple things after hospitalization. They forget to start a new medication. They stop an old medication by accident. The coordination that should happen—between doctor and hospital, between hospital and nursing home, between nursing home and home—doesn't happen. No one is watching the whole picture.

And then I see the nursing homes.

Seniors go to "skilled nursing facilities" to "get stronger" before they go home. That's what the system calls it. In reality, they go to be warehoused. I see patients who arrive alert and confused post-hospitalization, and within weeks they're zonked out on medications they didn't need, sedated into compliance, their minds fog-bound in a way we've all been trained to accept as "just aging."

It's not aging. It's too many medications. It's a system that extracts value at every turn—from the hospital that cuts nursing staff and discharges patients too early, from the insurance that denies safer alternatives, from the nursing home that medicates for convenience rather than necessity.

And we call it medicine.

This book exists because you deserve better. Your parent

deserves better. And the evidence to do better already exists.

The research is clear. The protocols work. The tools are available. What's missing is not knowledge. What's missing is someone saying: You don't have to accept this. You can see what's happening. You can intervene. You can demand better.

This book will teach you how.

It will show you how to see the prescribing cascade before it starts. How to talk to doctors in a way that maximizes their attention on your parent. How to coordinate care when the system won't. How to be the person in the room who understands the whole picture—because no one else will.

You will become a coordinator, a Conductor. You will manage the chaos that the system creates.

And when you're done with this book, you'll understand something deeper: the chaos isn't accidental. The system isn't broken by mistake. But understanding that becomes your cause for action.

Because systems designed for one purpose can be redirected by people who understand how they work.

Your parent's resilience got them this far. Now it's your turn to be resilient for them. To see clearly. To act with precision.

Read this book. Learn the tools. Use them.

The tightrope walker doesn't need to be in a hurricane. And neither does your parent.

In solidarity,

— **David Lee**
Portland, Oregon
Spring 2026

INTRODUCTION

The Well-Managed House

The kitchen counter has become a battlefield and you don't know how you got here.

On one side, there is a cluster of prescription bottles for your eighty-four-year-old mother, Barbara—a jumble of names you can't pronounce for conditions you don't fully understand. Next to them is a lineup of supplements you bought after reading an article online, their promised benefits a silent, hopeful prayer. Tucked in the corner is a weekly pill organizer, its rainbow-colored compartments a constant, stressful reminder of the complex regimen you are now responsible for managing.

This small patch of countertop is the epicenter of your new life, the physical manifestation of your role as an accidental caregiver in the "Sandwich Generation." It represents your deepest fears: a fear of making a mistake, a fear of what comes next for your mom, and the quiet, persistent fear that this cluttered chaos is a preview of your own future.

You look from her pillbox to your own reflection. You are fifty-five. You feel exhausted. Your own health has been relegated to the back burner, another task on a to-do list you never seem to reach. That persistent ache in your lower back, the way you walk into a room and forget why you're there—you dismiss these as normal signs of aging and stress. But in the quiet hours of the night, a more unsettling question bubbles to the surface: *Am I on the same path?*

Meanwhile, your senior black cat, Leo, watches the scene from his perch on a nearby chair, his gaze calm and inscrutable. At your feet, your old golden retriever, Sirius, lets out a soft sigh and rests his graying muzzle on your shoe, offering a simple, unconditional comfort that feels like the only sane thing in a world of medical complexity.

For years, I have seen this scene play out in a thousand different forms in my work as a geriatric pharmacist and former professor of geriatrics. I have sat with hundreds of people just like you, the accidental caregiver drowning in a sea of medical jargon, prescriptions, and well-intentioned but conflicting advice. They all share the same feeling of being overwhelmed, under-equipped, and profoundly alone.

Instead, I will show you how to find clarity, confidence, and even joy in your role by learning from the most unexpected teachers in your house: that stoic, observant cat and that loving, uncomplicated dog.

We look to them as guides not to diminish the profound dignity of your parent, but because our pet companions are masters of the non-verbal world. Beneath our complex human exterior, we share a fundamental mammalian nervous system that craves safety, comfort, and connection. By relearning this elemental language from them, we become better partners to the people we love.

Through their intuitive example, we will move toward the ultimate goal of this book: evolving from an

accidental caregiver to a true "care partner." Dr. Louise Aronson describes this critical transition from caregiver to care partner as acknowledging "a life-long human relationship. In a partnership, there is reciprocity. Even when a brain is changing, that person is still an active participant in their own life. To be a 'care partner' is to provide the support that allows the elder to remain a person, not a patient [1]." We will restore humanity through the haze of panic.

Together, we are going to explore a profound truth: the core principles of good care—keen observation, prioritizing function over lab results, ensuring safety, and providing comfort—are universal across species and ages. By learning to "read" the silent signals of your aging pet companions, you will become a better, more intuitive care partner for your parent. And in providing them with comfort, you will find the antidote to your own burnout.

Our guiding philosophy is simple: **Fewer Pills, More Paws**. This is not an anti-medication mantra. It is a commitment to using medications wisely and precisely, embracing the art of deprescribing—the safe reduction of unnecessary pills—to improve quality of life. And it is a recognition that sometimes the best medicine isn't a chemical, but a deeper connection to our companions who share our homes and our hearts.

Over the course of this book, you will be transformed. You will go from being an anxious, accidental caregiver to being the calm, confident conductor of your family's health orchestra. We will build, step-by-step, the systems you need to audit your mother's medicine cabinet, master the 8-minute doctor's appointment, and navigate the hardest conversations with grace. We will give you a "Longevity Toolkit" to manage your own health, ensuring you have the strength to lead for years to come with Barbara as your guide to, what I call, the *Path to the Pillbox* or the *Path to Fewer Pills, More Paws.*

The house may feel chaotic now, but it will become a well-managed house. Your fear will be replaced by knowledge, and your anxiety will be replaced by a profound sense of purpose. Let's begin.

PART 1 | THE BIOLOGY

The Health Profile of Your Full House

Before we can begin to manage a complex system, we must first understand its components. This first part of the book is a look at "why"—the fascinating and fundamental physiological changes that are shaping the health of every member of your household. It is our diagnostic phase. We are going to look under the hood of four very different but equally important biological systems: you, the fifty-five-year-old accidental caregiver; your eighty-four-year-old mother, Barbara; and your resident professors of physiology, Leo the cat and Sirius the dog.

We start with the body you know best: your own. From there, we'll turn to your mother's physiology before entering the surprising world of our pet companions. Let's take a tour of the fifty-five-year-old body, using science to find out why it feels different than it did at thirty. We will then demystify common frustrations, decode the "Overloaded Brain," and clearly lay out the two distinct paths—the *Path to the Pillbox* and the *Path to Fewer Pills, More Paws*—that diverge from this critical crossroads in your life.

After we understand your own body, we will take a tour of

our eighty-four-year-old body. Using science, we will reframe aging, seeing her body as a classic model with new requirements and specifications. We will learn the cause of many of the ailments of aging, **homeostenosis**, and establish the book's most important clinical philosophy: **prioritizing a person's daily function over a chase for perfect lab values**.

Finally, we will enter the surprising and fascinating world of our pet companions. By exploring the unique anatomy and metabolism of cats and dogs, we will learn lessons about medication safety, individuality, and the wisdom that "less is more"—lessons that apply directly to the human members of our full house.

By the end of this section, you will see your family's health not as a series of random, frightening problems, but as an interconnected system governed by understandable rules. This knowledge is the foundation upon which all your newfound confidence and skill will be built.

1 | THE 55-YEAR-OLD AT THE CROSSROADS

Your Body's 'New-ish' Owner's Manual and the Two Paths Ahead

Does it feel like the rules have changed and you're not sure when?

Maybe you strode confidently to the living room to get...something—if only you could remember. Or the unwelcome groan or click your body makes when you stand up from a low chair. Perhaps it's the quiet frustration of looking in the mirror and seeing a stranger who seems to be holding onto weight in places it never used to stick. You haven't changed the fundamentals—you're still *you*—but it feels as though the body you've known for decades has been swapped out for a similar, yet more finicky, model. The new owner's manual, it seems, is written in a language you don't quite understand, and no one ever handed it to you.

If this sounds familiar, I understand all too well: You are not alone, you are not imagining it, and you are not failing. Based on decades of research that is finally changing how we view middle age, you are standing at one of the most significant physiological crossroads of your life. This isn't just a slow slide into "old age." Welcome to middle age—a distinct and fascinating biological state with its own set of rules [1].

You see a reflection of this crossroads most clearly when you look at your own aging parent. You stand in the kitchen with your eighty-four-year-old mother, Barbara, and watch her meticulously sort her weekly pill organizer—a rainbow of tablets for blood pressure, cholesterol, bone density, and sleep. You see the path she is on, what I call *The Path to the Pillbox*, and a quiet dread settles in your chest. *Is that my future?*

You can avoid the overflowing pillbox but avoiding it requires understanding the new owner's manual. This chapter *is* that manual. We are going to take a detailed, head-to-toe tour of the fifty-five-year-old body, explaining *why* it feels different than it did at thirty, especially if you're also experiencing menopause. We'll look at the hard science, but we'll translate it into plain English. More importantly, we're going to illuminate the two paths that diverge from this very spot: the *Path to the Pillbox*, like Barbara's overflowing pillbox, and the *Path to Fewer Pills, More Paws*, which leads to a longer, healthier, more vital life. The choice begins with the century's old mantra: *Know Thyself.*

A Tour of your Fifty-five-Year-Old Body

Think of your body at thirty, or you may have kids close to this age. It was likely a highly resilient machine. It had a wide, forgiving margin for error. You could probably still push it—a stressful work week, a few nights of poor sleep—and bounce back with relative ease. Your physiology could absorb insults and errors with little protest.

At fifty-five, that buffer zone has narrowed; the margin for error is less. Your body is still capable, but it's less forgiving of neglect. The bill for poor decisions now comes due much more quickly with a bigger toll. Let's explore your body, system by system.

Perimenopause and Menopause

If men are easing into middle age, women are experiencing middle age with terrifying intensity. Between 45 and 55, women experience a specific biological hurricane complicating nearly every system in the middle-aged body: **Perimenopause and Menopause.**

For decades, estrogen has kept your body resilient and flexible. It was a systemic protector. It kept your arteries flexible. It protected your brain's processing speed. It maintained your bone density. It helped regulate your insulin.

As we go through each system, we will point out how menopause is intensifying the journey into middle age.

Your Heart

One of the most profound, yet completely silent, changes happening inside you right now is within your miles of blood vessels. The elastic, responsive arteries of your past are gradually, but predictably, becoming stiffer.

When you were younger, your major arteries, especially the aorta, were rich in a wonderfully flexible protein called **elastin**. This allowed them to expand easily with every heartbeat, smoothing out the pressure wave. Starting around age thirty, however, a structural shift begins. Like an old rubber band, the elastin fibers begin to fray and degrade. In their place, your body deposits a tougher, more fibrous protein called **collagen** [2]. This process, **arteriosclerosis**, is a universal feature of vascular aging. Collagen provides strength, but it lacks flexibility.

At thirty, this stiffening process was underway, but it was largely invisible. Your blood pressure was likely still in a healthy range. But in the twenty-five years since, that slow replacement of elastin with collagen has reached a tipping point. The change is no longer subtle.

No doubt you've heard the analogy of blood pressure to water pressure in a garden hose. A new garden hose is still quite flexible. When you turn on the spigot, its walls expand slightly to handle the surge, and the stream is smooth and even. Now, imagine that same hose after another 2-3 years in the sun and cold. It's rigid. When you turn on the same spigot with the same force, the hose doesn't yield; the pressure inside spikes violently. Eventually, cracks will form. They are small at first, but have no doubt: the walls are weakening. At fifty-five, your arteries are stiffer. Your heart is pushing blood into a container that no longer yields. To move blood through this stiffer circuit, your blood pressure must rise.

For women, estrogen was helping keep your arteries distinctively elastic. When estrogen leaves, vascular aging accelerates. This is why a woman's risk of heart disease catches up to men's within a decade of menopause.

This slow, steady stiffening is why **hypertension** is an epidemic in middle age. You don't feel your arteries getting harder. The first sign is often a high number on a blood pressure cuff during a routine check-up: 145/90 mmHg. Your doctor expresses concern. If it remains elevated, the standard medical response is swift: a prescription for a diuretic like hydrochlorothiazide. For women, this may be 10 years after men, but menopause quickly accelerates the need for the diuretic. The pill works by reducing the fluid volume in your stiff hose, lowering the pressure. Just like that, you've taken your first step onto the *Path to the Pillbox*. The issue isn't the pill itself; it's an elegant fix for the immediate pressure problem. The issue is that if it is ignored it will lead to predictable symptoms. Those cracks get filled in with cholesterol, a weak spot in the wall of the vessel. Blood pressure medications are amazing miracles that have reduced strokes in half since introduced. There is a reason hypertension medications are the number one daily medications for middle-aged adults. But the *Path to Fewer Pills, More Paws* is built on lifestyle choices that achieve these same results, where the only side effect is better health.

Your Muscles, Bones, and Joints

That new ache in your knee, or the surprising effort it took to lift that heavy bag of potting soil isn't just a random event. It's a symptom of a fundamental shift in your body's architecture—a process that has been silently at work since you blew out your thirtieth birthday candles.

The term for this is **sarcopenia**, the slow, age-related theft of our muscle mass and function [3]. While it begins in our thirties, its effects become undeniable in our fifties. We can lose 3-8% of our muscle mass per decade, and the rate accelerates after age sixty [4]. This is driven by hormonal changes and by a state of "anabolic resistance," where your muscles become less responsive to the protein you eat, making it harder to build new tissue.

At thirty, you likely still felt physically robust. Sarcopenia had begun, but its effects were largely imperceptible. You could play hard on the weekend and bounce back. At fifty-five, the *cumulative effect* of fifteen years of this slow, quiet theft makes itself known. Your muscle mass, the powerful "shock absorbers" for your skeleton, is measurably smaller. This means more force from walking and lifting is transferred directly to your joints, which is why your knees or your back are "achier." Your muscles, which act as giant metabolic "sponges" for blood sugar, are also smaller, making it harder to manage your weight. This isn't a sudden failure; it's the revealing of a process that's been underway for years.

Let's imagine your eleven-year-old golden retriever, Sirius. When he was younger, he'd leap off the bed with a single bound. Now, you notice he slides off gently. He doesn't bolt for the door; he rises slowly and performs an elaborate, full-body stretch, elongating his spine and legs with a groan. He isn't being lazy; he's being wise. He is instinctively honoring the stiffness in his aging joints and the diminished shock absorption from his muscles. That preparatory stretch is his non-negotiable ritual for a day of pain-free function. He is showing you, not telling you, that his body has new rules. This is a lesson in observation we will come back to again and again.

Menopause especially speeds up muscle loss. This is an area that women must pay particular attention to avoid the physical frailty that can lead to a hip fracture or to even be bed bound in profound cases.

Sarcopenia is a direct route to the medicine cabinet. Achy joints lead to reaching for NSAIDs like ibuprofen (Advil/Motrin) more often. Less muscle and a slower metabolism are a primary cause of weight gain and rising blood sugar. At your physical, your doctor notes your elevated cholesterol and blood sugar. A prescription for a statin or a pre-diabetes drug like metformin isn't far behind. You've now added two or three more bottles and another step down the *Path to the Pillbox.*

Your Metabolism, Liver, and Fat

"I eat the same way I always have, but I keep gaining weight." This is one of the most common and demoralizing refrains of middle age. It is not a failure of willpower. It is a predictable change in your metabolic engine.

The combination of losing metabolically active muscle tissue and a natural slowdown in cellular activity means your basal metabolic rate declines. At the same time, your body's cells often become less sensitive to the hormone **insulin** [5]. Your pancreas has to work harder, pumping out more insulin to get sugar into your cells. High insulin levels are a powerful signal to your body to store fat, particularly inflammatory **visceral fat** around your internal organs. Meanwhile, your liver, the master chemical processing plant, is a little slower at its job, just like a processing plant that's been running daily for decades.

At thirty, your metabolism was still a relatively steady fire. You had more wiggle room. By fifty-five, the fire has banked to a slower, cooler burn. It doesn't need as much fuel, and if you give it the same amount you did at thirty, the excess just piles up.

Think of your cat, Leo. He is a master of listening to his body. If his food isn't fresh, he sniffs it with disdain and walks away. His system is highly specialized, and he instinctively rejects anything that isn't optimal for him. Our human bodies send us similar signals all the time when they're not getting the right fuel—indigestion, bloating, fatigue. In our busy lives, we've just gotten exceptionally good at taking an antacid and powering through.

This metabolic shift is the direct on-ramp to two of the most common prescriptions on the planet: statins and diabetes medications. When your bloodwork comes back with elevated LDL cholesterol, high triglycerides, and a fasting glucose in the pre-diabetic range, the medical response is clear and evidence-based. These pills are effective, but they are treating the symptoms of metabolic changes going on at this point for years.

Your Kidneys

While the changes to your kidneys are subtle, they play a crucial role in your health and, critically, your tolerance for medications.

Kidney function naturally declines with normal healthy aging. One of the most important consequences is that your kidneys become less adept at handling large loads of **sodium** [6]. Your body becomes more "salt-sensitive," meaning the same amount of dietary salt will raise your blood pressure more than it would have when you were younger.

At thirty, your kidneys could flush out the sodium from a large bag of potato chips with relative ease. At fifty-five, after eating that same bag, your less-efficient kidneys struggle to keep up. More sodium and the water that follows it are retained in your bloodstream, increasing the pressure in your stiff garden hose.

This increased salt sensitivity is another key contributor to hypertension. Understanding this simple physiological fact—that your body's relationship with salt has changed—is a profoundly empowering piece of knowledge for taking control of your health. Otherwise, we might not be aware of how "a little salt" is helping to put cracks in the garden hose. It will not cause immediate failure, but this is how the aging process works: accumulating small cracks over a lifetime.

Your Overloaded Brain

This is the big one. For me, and for many of my patients, this is the change that sparks the most fear. You walk into a room and forget why. A common word is suddenly out of reach. You worry, *Is this the beginning of the end? Am I getting dementia?*

The data suggests this is likely a functional state, not a disease state. What you are likely experiencing is not a disease. It is a temporary, functional state I call **The Overloaded Brain.**

Your brain at fifty-five is not "failing." It is chronically and profoundly overloaded. This load, the stressors of life, and all the things you must remember at any given time is called Cognitive Load. Your brain has a finite capacity, there are only so many things your exquisite brain can do at once. This capacity is called Cognitive Reserve. Groceries, kids, bills, remembering to walk Sirius, lunch, sleep, laundry, litter box, and what are you going to make for dinner? On top of all that, Barbara has fallen, her neighbor tells you over the phone. The Cognitive Load has exceeded your Cognitive Reserve. Welcome to The Overloaded Brain. Managing the health of aging parents, navigating more complex finances, thinking about retirement, and dealing with your own hormonal shifts are not unique to middle age but maybe they seem more prescient at this time.

Estrogen receptors are dense in the hippocampus, responsible for memory, and prefrontal cortex, responsible for focus. When estrogen drops during menopause, those neurons temporarily misfire. That "brain fog" you feel isn't just because you are busy; it is a withdrawal symptom from a powerful neuroprotective hormone.

On top of this, you are layering on two physiological disruptors. First, the chronic, low-grade stress elevates the hormone **cortisol**, which can directly interfere with the function of the hippocampus, the brain region critical for forming new memories [7]. Second, the notoriously poor sleep of middle age prevents the brain from performing its essential nightly "clean-up cycle," where it clears out metabolic debris and consolidates memories [8].

For women during menopause, the drop in progesterone devastates women's sleep; progesterone helped to calm the nervous system. The drop in progesterone and the thermal chaos of hot flashes destroy sleep quality. This exacerbates "The Overloaded Brain," making you feel less resilient.

At thirty, your brain was busy. At fifty-five, your brain is just as busy but your brain isn't as plastic as before, meaning it's not as adaptable. You are exchanging flexibility for crystallized intelligence. **Crystallized intelligence** represents the deep reservoir of knowledge, patterns, and wisdom that you have accumulated over a lifetime of experience. Unlike physical brain volume or processing speed which may decline in healthy aging, this type of intelligence is remarkably well-preserved during healthy aging. Physically, this may be represented by the quality of synaptic connections between brain cells or regions, maintaining flexibility and wisdom. It contributes to your cognitive reserve, allowing your brain to maintain function by rerouting neural traffic through these established connections even as physical changes occur. Remarkably, your brain becomes faster at certain tasks, those that have taken a lifetime to learn.

As remarkable as your brain is, it's often on too little restorative sleep and bathed in a sea of low-grade stress hormones. It is not failing; it is just hitting its cognitive limit. The occasional "glitch"—like a forgotten name—is a symptom of this overload, not a sign of dementia. It's a yellow warning light on your dashboard, not an engine seizure.

This is one of the most important concepts in this book. By reframing your forgetfulness from a terrifying sign of disease to a manageable, functional issue of an overloaded system, we take away the fear. Fear is paralyzing. Taking away the fear allows you to act. The solution isn't a pill or supplement for dementia; it's a proactive strategy to address the root causes: managing stress, prioritizing sleep, and jettisoning the destructive myth of multitasking. Investing in the *Path to Fewer Pills, More Paws* is an investment that pays dividends. You get a brain that is clearer, better able to handle the challenges of the day.

Sometimes, the best action is surprisingly simple. Think of your cat, Leo. When you sit down, vibrating with the stress of the day, he jumps into your lap, settles his weight onto your chest, and begins to purr. It isn't just comforting; it is medicinal. Studies have suggested that the frequency of a cat's purr—between 25 and 150 Hz—corresponds to vibrational frequencies that can lower blood pressure and decrease stress hormones. Leo is dispensing a potent, biologically active anti-anxiety treatment with zero negative side effects. We can't bottle a purr, but we can recognize that the path to a calmer brain often lies in simple, natural connection rather than a prescription.

That's not the only way Leo teaches you to be the Zen master. The "Slow Blink"—the way Leo closes his eyes for one second while looking at you—signals calmness and acceptance. For a predator like Leo, staring is a threat. Their slow blink is regarding you with trust, and for a lean mean predator, that's a lot. His slow blink is his version of a hug.

Leo has another neurochemical way of relaxing you. Studies have shown that petting and playing with cats releases Oxytocin, the love hormone. It is a bio-feedback loop usually reserved for mother-infant bonding.

As impressive as Leo is, Sirius is the true master of this hack. When you stare into Sirius's eyes, both of your brains are flooded with oxytocin, up to 300% more. While Sirius stares into your eyes to release love, Leo does it by demanding that scratch on his back and by pouncing on that string you dangle for him. When Leo is giving you that nudge on your elbow demanding attention, he is demanding a deeper level of connection with you. He is offering you some anti-anxiety.

Understanding the "Window of Opportunity" for Hormone Replacement Therapy

At this crossroads, you will likely face a decision your mother didn't have the luxury of understanding clearly: Hormone

Replacement Therapy (HRT).

For twenty years, women were terrified of HRT. In 2002, a massive study called the Women's Health Initiative (WHI) was abruptly stopped because it showed increased risks of breast cancer and stroke. Overnight, millions of women flushed their pills, and doctors stopped prescribing them.

But we missed a critical detail: The women in that study were, on average, 63 years old. Many had already gone without estrogen for a decade.

The 2022 position statement of the North American Menopause Society (NAMS) supports initiating hormone therapy in healthy women within ten years of menopause onset, when the benefits for most women outweigh the risks.

If you are healthy and start HRT within 10 years of menopause, the window is still open for you, the benefits often outweigh the risks. Estrogen can help keep your still-flexible arteries soft, protect your bone density, and clear the "brain fog" by stabilizing neural networks. It is a powerful tool for extending your healthspan.

If you wait until you are Barbara's age to start, the door has likely closed. We will discuss why in the next chapter.

Do not suffer in silence because of old headlines. If you are struggling with sleep, brain fog, or hot flashes, find a menopause-certified practitioner. You are likely in the window where this is not just safe, but protective.

Your Choice at the Crossroads

And so, here you are, suddenly fifty-five. You now understand that the slight rise in blood pressure, the achy knees, and The Overloaded Brain are not random failures but predictable outcomes of a system entering a new phase. Now you can clearly see the two paths stretching out before you.

The *Path to the Pillbox*

This is the path of least resistance. You don't make any major changes. You accept the aches and fatigue as inevitable. You treat the symptoms as they arise, one by one. The high blood pressure reading gets a diuretic. The high cholesterol gets a statin. The achy joints get daily NSAIDs. Before you know it, you are seventy, and your medicine cabinet looks exactly like Barbara's. You have amassed yourself a collection of side effects from a collection of pills, a condition called **polypharmacy**. This is the passive, default path. We are all headed down it whether we are ready or not.

The *Path to Fewer Pills, More Paws*

This path requires a choice. It is a path of engagement, not perfection. It is built on the knowledge you've just gained.

It acknowledges that if your arteries are stiffening, the answer lies not just in a pill, but in movement that improves flexibility and a diet that reduces inflammation. It accepts that if you're losing muscle, the solution is targeted strength training and adequate protein. It understands that if your brain is overloaded, the remedy is radical self-care: prioritizing sleep and managing stress.

This path is about giving your body what its fifty-five-year-old brain truly needs. And sometimes, the best way to do that is to look to the simple wisdom in your own home—the uncomplicated companionship of a dog like Sirius, the quiet lesson in mindfulness from a cat like Leo.

Sirius doesn't care that you are tired, stressed, or busy. He needs a walk. That simple, non-negotiable demand forces you out of your head and into your body. It forces you into fresh air and movement. Science backs up what Sirius knows instinctively: dog owners have been shown to have lower blood pressure, better cholesterol levels, and a reduced risk of heart disease compared to non-owners, largely because that leash forces us to keep moving. While the *Path to the Pillbox* is often sedentary, the *Path to Fewer Pills, More Paws* is inherently active, guided by a companion who knows that movement is life.

This is not a story of inevitable decline. It is a story of a choice that stands before you today. You now have the map. And to fully understand where the *Path to the Pillbox* leads and why the *Path to Fewer Pills, More Paws* is so vital, we must first truly understand the world your parent inhabits. Let's turn the page and look at the world through Barbara's eighty-four-year-old eyes.

Why the 84-Year-Old Body Requires a Master's Touch

We just took an honest look at our own fifty-five-year-old bodies. We reframed those frustrating memory lapses not as a terrifying sign of decline, but as a manageable symptom of The Overloaded Brain.

Now, we must turn our attention to the other side of the care partnership: your eighty-four-year-old mother, Barbara.

You look at her and see the woman who raised you, a person layered with a lifetime of memories, strength, and love. But her physical reality is now profoundly different from your own, and worlds away from what it was when she was thirty.

To care for her well—to be her best advocate and her most compassionate partner—we must first become fluent in the sheet music of her body's new composition.

It's tempting to view aging through a lens of decay, as if the eighty-four-year-old body is just a broken-down version of a younger one. But I will offer you a different view: **Barbara's body is not a failing machine; she is a Stradivarius violin.** Stradivarius violins were crafted by Antonio Stradivari in Cremona, Italy, around 1700. These violins are considered the finest ever made. Today, a single one can sell for over $15 million, and scientists still cannot perfectly replicate their sound.

She is a vintage masterpiece, built with decades of resilience. But like a fine, aged instrument, she has become **temperamental**. As Louise Aronson notes in 'Elderhood,' we are simply navigating a distinct life stage [1]. A Stradivarius isn't 'failing' because it's old; it's transitioning into a state of **higher sensitivity**. We need to stop treating aging as a disease to be cured and start treating it as a stage to be lived.

She needs a different kind of care, a more attentive musician, and a profound respect for her fragility. If you understand how to tune this instrument, she can still play beautiful music.

This chapter is your guide to that instrument.

Geriatric Physiology

If you learn only one new medical term from this book, let it be this one: **homeostenosis**.

It sounds complicated, but the concept is profoundly simple and critically important. *Homeo* refers to homeostasis, the body's remarkable ability to maintain a stable internal environment—like a thermostat keeping your house at a steady temperature. *Stenosis* is a Greek root meaning a narrowing. Therefore, homeostenosis is the progressive, age-related **narrowing of our physiological buffer zones** [2].

Let's use a tightrope walker analogy. A thirty-year-old has the luxury of walking on a wide, forgiving platform. If they get hit by a gust of wind—like a minor infection, feel a bit dehydrated from a busy day, or have a poor night's sleep—they have plenty of room to wobble, correct their balance, and continue on without danger. Their buffer zone is wide.

Barbara, at eighty-four, is walking on a rope that is just as strong, but it has become a very narrow tightrope. Her body, when it is at rest and unchallenged, can maintain perfect balance. Her blood pressure is stable, her temperature is normal, her blood sugar is in range. But when she is hit by the very same gust of wind on that tight rope—the same common cold, the same missed glass of water, a new medication—her capacity to wobble is gone. She has almost no buffer zone. A minor disturbance doesn't just cause a wobble on the tight rope; it can trigger a catastrophic fall.

This single concept explains almost every crisis in geriatric medicine.

It's why a simple urinary tract infection in a thirty-year-old is an annoyance, but in an eighty-four-year-old, it can cause acute delirium and hospitalization.

It's why a bout of the stomach flu might make a younger person miserable for a day, but for Barbara, the resulting dehydration and electrolyte imbalance could lead to acute kidney failure and a dangerous fall.

It's why a standard adult dose of a common sleep aid can leave an older adult confused and "hungover" for a full day.

Understanding homeostenosis is the knowledge and power to predict. It shifts your mindset from reacting to major problems to proactively preventing the minor disturbances that *cause* the major problems. It teaches you that in caring for a classic model, small details are everything. With that golden rule firmly in mind, let's begin our head-to-toe tour.

A Tour of the Eighty-four-Year-Old Body

The Eighty-four-Year-Old Heart

The aging heart is a testament to endurance, having beaten

over three billion times by age eighty-four. It is a powerful organ, but it is not the same nimble, responsive heart it was at thirty.

Over decades, the heart muscle itself remodels. The walls of the left ventricle, the main pumping chamber, thicken and stiffen in a process called **left ventricular hypertrophy** [3]. The muscle becomes less compliant, meaning the chamber doesn't relax as easily to fill with blood between beats, this is called diastolic dysfunction. The valves that control blood flow can become calcified and stiff, known as valvular sclerosis. The heart's own internal "pacemaker" system, the sinoatrial node, can lose cells, and its sensitivity to adrenaline—the hormone that tells the heart to speed up—diminishes. This means the aged heart has a lower maximum achievable heart rate.

At thirty, the heart was an athletic organ. When you sprinted for a bus, your heart rate could leap from 70 to 160 beats per minute in seconds, dramatically increasing cardiac output. At eighty-four, Barbara's heart is a strong, dependable workhorse, but not a racehorse. Its resting function is excellent, but its ability to respond to stress—its "cardiac reserve"—is significantly reduced. When faced with a demand like climbing a flight of stairs, her heart rate might only climb from 70 to 110 bpm. It cannot ramp up as quickly or as high. This isn't a sign of disease; it's a normal feature of the aged heart.

A healthy, active eighty-four-year-old has, through consistent exercise, maintained a more efficient cardiovascular system. They can still climb that flight of stairs, though they'll be breathing more heavily. In a frail individual, this diminished reserve is much more pronounced. The simple act of standing up can be a cardiovascular challenge, sometimes leading to **orthostatic hypotension**—a sudden drop in blood pressure that causes dizziness and is a major cause of falls.

You must respect this diminished reserve. Rushing an older adult is not just frustrating for them; it's physiologically stressful. It's like asking the 30-year-old body to run a 400-meter dash with no training over and over again. This is also where medications become critical. Many blood pressure medications, particularly those that dilate blood vessels, can worsen orthostatic hypotension. It's crucial to monitor Barbara for dizziness upon standing, especially after a new medication or dose change is introduced.

The Eighty-four-Year-Old Kidneys

If there is one system that dictates the rules of geriatric pharmacology, it is the kidneys. Their age-related changes are predictable, profound, and have massive implications for medication safety.

As we age, the total mass of our kidneys decreases. More importantly, the number of functioning filtration units, called **nephrons**, declines, and the blood vessels supplying the kidneys can harden. The result is a steady, predictable decline in the **glomerular filtration rate (GFR)**, the best measure of kidney function. By age eighty, the GFR can be reduced by 30-50% compared to a young adult, even in someone with no diagnosed kidney disease [4]. This is a normal, non-pathological part of aging.

The kidneys of a thirty-year-old are powerhouses of filtration. They have a massive functional reserve. If they take an NSAID like ibuprofen, their kidneys clear it swiftly. If they become slightly dehydrated, their kidneys skillfully concentrate urine to conserve every last drop of water. At eighty-four, Barbara's kidneys are still working diligently, but with half the workforce and less robust plumbing. Their ability to clear medications from the blood is significantly slowed. That same dose of ibuprofen now lingers in her system for much longer, increasing the risk of acute kidney injury. Due to homeostenosis, her ability to handle dehydration or electrolyte shifts is also severely impaired.

> **♀ Pharmacist Pro Tip! ♀**
>
> Always drink plenty of water when taking an NSAID. They squeeze the arteries going to the kidneys. If your parent is dehydrated, the amount of blood getting to their kidneys is a trickle. Dehydration is one of the biggest threats to the long-term health of their kidneys—and yours.

Think back to Leo. Cats' kidneys are desert-adapted super-concentrators, making them prone to burning out over time. While human kidneys are different, the lesson is the same: a critical filtration system under a lifetime of strain becomes vulnerable. The reduced function in Barbara's kidneys is not a disease; it is the predictable result of eighty-four years of dedicated continuous service with no breaks.

This is paramount for medication safety. **Because of reduced kidney clearance, a standard adult dose of many common medications can effectively be a toxic overdose for an eighty-four-year-old.** This applies to everything from certain antibiotics (like ciprofloxacin), diabetes medications (like metformin), heart medications (like digoxin), to over-the-counter pain relievers (like NSAIDs). This is why the pharmacist's mantra is "start low, go slow" in older adults. Any medication cleared by the kidneys—and there are hundreds—requires careful dose consideration for Barbara.

The Eighty-four-Year-Old Liver

The liver is the body's other great chemical processing factory. Like the kidneys, its function also changes with age, though in a different manner.

The key changes are a reduction in the liver's total mass and, more importantly, a significant decrease in the amount of blood flowing to it—by as much as 40% [5]. This is critical for drugs that are typically cleared very quickly by the liver on their "first pass" after being absorbed from the gut. With less blood flow, less of the drug is removed before it reaches the rest of the body. This effectively increases the **bioavailability**—the amount of active drug that reached the circulation—of many common medications. Ironically, the slowed blood flow doesn't matter for moderately cleared drugs by the liver. To say the least, it's complicated.

At thirty, the liver is a large organ with robust blood flow. It efficiently processes nutrients and metabolizes medications, acting as a powerful buffer with extra capacity. At eighty-four, Barbara's liver is smaller, and the blood flowing to it is much slower and less voluminous. While the enzymatic active components are still competent, they just don't get as much raw material delivered to them as quickly.

If the fifty-five-year-old liver is a chemical processing factory that has slowed down, this is even more true for Barbara. The chemical factory takes longer and its capacity is limited. Thus, it's easier to overwhelm its capacity. It's much easier to be overloaded with multiple medications at once; the chemical plant just cannot handle all the chemicals at once.

This is the other half of the drug-safety equation. Certain medications, including some opioids, beta-blockers, benzodiazepines, and antidepressants, can have a much more powerful effect in Barbara because of this reduced clearance. This reinforces the need for lower starting doses and careful monitoring. It's also why adding even a seemingly benign herbal supplement can be risky—it's one more item being tossed into that slowed down chemical processing factory.

The Eighty-four-Year-Old Muscles

We introduced sarcopenia in Chapter 1, but in the context of an eighty-four-year-old, it becomes one of the central dramas of aging, setting the stage for the dreaded condition of frailty.

Sarcopenia is now in its advanced stages. There is not just a loss of muscle mass, but a preferential loss of the powerful, fast-twitch Type II muscle fibers, which are responsible for rapid movements like catching one's balance. The slower, endurance-focused Type I fibers are better preserved [6]. This is why older adults lose *power*—the ability to generate force quickly—even more dramatically than they lose raw strength.

This loss of power creates a vicious downward spiral, often called the **"Frailty Cycle"** [7]. Sarcopenia leads to a slower walking speed and weakness. This weakness makes physical activity difficult, leading to even more inactivity. Inactivity accelerates muscle loss and lowers the metabolic rate. This often leads to a decreased appetite and poor nutrition, which further exacerbates muscle wasting. The cycle continues, leading to frailty, falls, and a loss of independence.

This is where the path of the healthy ager and the frail individual diverge most dramatically. A healthy, non-frail eighty-four-year-old has actively fought against this cycle with resistance exercise and a protein-rich diet. A frail individual is one who has been caught in the cycle and now meets the clinical criteria: *unintentional weight loss, self-reported exhaustion, weakness (measured by grip strength), slow walking speed, and low physical activity.*

For Barbara, preventing and combating this cycle is a top priority. Every bit of functional independence she has depends on the strength left in her muscles. Your role as a care partner is to be a champion for her strength: encouraging gentle exercise, preparing protein-rich meals, and, critically, reviewing her medications for any that might cause weakness or sedation and thus accelerate the frailty cycle.

The Eighty-four-Year-Old Gut

The digestive system, from top to bottom, undergoes a variety of changes that can impact nutrition and comfort.

Saliva production often decreases, leading to dry mouth (xerostomia), which makes chewing and swallowing difficult and increases the risk of dental cavities. In the stomach, production of gastric acid can decline (atrophic gastritis), which can impair the absorption of certain nutrients that require an acidic environment, most notably Vitamin B_{12}, calcium, and iron [8]. The entire GI tract's motility slows down, a major contributor to **constipation**.

At thirty, the GI tract is resilient and efficient. At eighty-four, Barbara's GI tract is more sensitive and operates at a slower pace. The dry mouth may be exacerbated by many common medications, like diuretics or antidepressants. The reduced acid may mean she isn't getting the full benefit from her food or supplements. The slow motility means she is in a constant battle against constipation, a condition that can be miserable and is a primary cause of delirium if severe.

This means for your mom, you become a "gut detective." Is Mom's new confusion related to a Vitamin B12 deficiency? Is her constipation a side effect of her pain medication? Or a little of both? Encouraging fluid intake, a fiber-rich diet, and regular movement are non-negotiable first-line strategies. This is a classic example of where "fewer pills" is the goal— resolving medication-induced constipation is far better than adding a daily laxative to the pillbox. As a pharmacist, I've seen many older adults needing surgery for fecal impaction–that's how serious this can be.

The Eighty-four-Year-Old Immune System
One of the most exciting frontiers in gerontology is our understanding of the aging immune system. The changes are twofold: the system becomes less effective at fighting off new invaders, and it gets stuck in a state of chronic, low-grade activation.

The ability to mount a swift, robust response to new pathogens or to vaccines declines with age, a process called **immunosenescence**. This is partly due to the shrinking of the thymus, the gland responsible for maturing our elite T-cells [9]. At the same time, the aging body exists in a state of chronic, low-level inflammation, a phenomenon dubbed **"inflammaging"** [10]. This background "noise" of inflammation is now thought to be a major driver of many age-related chronic diseases, from atherosclerosis to Alzheimer's disease.

At thirty, the immune system is in its prime. It reacts fiercely to infection and then quiets down. At eighty-four, Barbara's immune system is like an old, weary guard. It's slower to recognize a new threat, allowing infections to gain a foothold. And it's constantly quietly screaming to itself with inflammaging, which contributes to her joint pain.

This is why "a little cold" can be a very big deal for Barbara. Infection prevention is a top priority. This means zealous attention to handwashing, avoiding crowds during flu season, and ensuring she is up to date on all recommended vaccinations, such as influenza, pneumonia, RSV, COVID-19, and shingles. These are critical acts as a care partner.

♀ Pharmacist Pro Tip! ♀

Recent clinical studies showed the Shingrix™ (shingles) and Arexvy™ (RSV) vaccine reduces the risk of dementia by up to 20% [11].

The Eighty-four-Year-Old Brain

The changes in the eighty-four-year-old brain are different from the "Overloaded Brain" of middle age and relate to the physical hardware itself.

With age, there is some inevitable loss of brain volume and synaptic connections. This results in slower processing speeds; however, intelligence is maintained well into later life. Additionally, crystallized intelligence is remarkably well-preserved in healthy aging. The key concept here is **cognitive**

reserve, the brain's ability to find alternative routes or workarounds when one neural pathway is damaged. A person who has spent their life learning and staying engaged has a high cognitive reserve [12]. In other words, an active and engaged brain has more synaptic connections to maintain memory, make new memories, and remember life-long skills. When age-related changes begin to damage some connections, their brain can reroute traffic, maintaining function for longer.

Your role is to protect the magnificent library that is Barbara's mind. This means reducing the cognitive load. Routine is calming and essential. Instructions should be simple and broken down into single steps. Most importantly, you must protect her brain from chemical insults—this means relentlessly vetting her medication list for anything that can cause confusion or sedation (the anticholinergics, the benzodiazepines) and working with her doctor to find alternatives.

The Eighty-four-Year-Old Skin

Changes in the skin have major implications for health and safety.

The skin's outer layer, the **epidermis**, thins, and the connection to the layer beneath, the **dermis**, becomes more fragile. The subcutaneous fat layer, which provides cushioning, also thins dramatically. Sweat and oil gland function decreases, leading to dried cracked skin [13].

The skin at thirty is thick and resilient. At eighty-four, Barbara's skin is like tissue paper. A minor bump can cause a large bruise (senile purpura). Medical tape can tear the skin.

The lack of fat makes her more sensitive to cold and increases her risk of developing pressure ulcers.

Gentle is the watchword. This means gentle handling, using moisturizer liberally, and checking for red spots over bony areas like her tailbone or heels. It also impacts medication: transdermal patches may not adhere as well and can cause more irritation.

The skin serves as the primary interface for safety and comfort for everyone in the room, but its sensitivity varies dramatically. For Barbara, the skin has become thinner and more fragile, like tissue paper, losing the protective layer of subcutaneous fat that once provided cushioning. This makes her more sensitive to cold and pressure, meaning a touch that feels firm to you might feel sharp or bruising to her, requiring a gentle, deliberate approach to avoid injury.

Your pets use touch as a robust communication tool that bypasses their conscious brains. Sirius responds to deep pressure therapy—a firm hug or a tight "thundershirt"—which bypasses his frantic brain during a storm to mechanically trigger his calming parasympathetic nervous system. Leo retains a primal connection to touch from kittenhood, often "kneading" blankets to release oxytocin and signal safety. While Barbara's skin requires protection, she shares this fundamental mammalian need for comforting, rhythmic touch to feel safe.

The Eighty-four-Year-Old Eyes and Ears

The way Barbara experiences the world is different, as the portals of information—her eyes and ears—undergo predictable changes.

In the eye, the lens becomes stiffer (presbyopia) and yellows. The pupil becomes smaller and less responsive to light, impairing night vision. In the ear, the loss of sensory hair cells leads to age-related hearing loss (presbycusis), which particularly affects the ability to hear high-frequency consonants such as "s" or "f", making it hard to distinguish words.

You must be her amplifier and magnifier. Ensure prescriptions have large-print labels. Speak clearly and face-to-face. Understand that if she doesn't respond, it's not because she is ignoring you; she very likely did not hear you. Recognizing this sensory barrier is a profound act of empathy.

🔎 Pharmacist Pro Tip! 🔎

Your pharmacist can provide instructions in an alternative form, such as an audio recording or large print (or language)—just ask. Under the Americans with Disabilities Act (ADA) and the Affordable Care Act, pharmacies are required to provide accessible information (like large print or translation) to ensure you understand your medication.

The visual and auditory worlds of your household are split between those who see detail and those who see motion. You and Barbara are trichromatic, perceiving the rich world of Red, Green, and Blue, which allows you to appreciate art and subtle emotional cues. Leo and Sirius live in a dichromatic world, blind to Red and Green, seeing your home in washed-out shades of blue and yellow. However, they possess a visual superpower that you lack. Their eyes refresh images significantly faster than yours, allowing them to detect microscopic movements—like the twitch of a mouse or a leaf falling—that your brain completely misses. Leo complements this with ultrasonic hearing that reaches 64,000 Hz, compared to your 20,000 Hz limit, effectively wiring him to hear the heartbeat of prey inside a wall while you are straining to hear the television.

Why the HRT Window Has Closed

You might wonder: *If estrogen is so protective for the brain and bones, why don't we just put Barbara on it now?*

This is the other side of the "Timing Hypothesis."

Remember the "stiff garden hose" analogy? By age 84, Barbara's arteries have stiffened and likely have some silent plaque buildup. This is normal aging.

If we reintroduce systemic estrogen now, after decades without it, it acts differently than it did when she was 55. Instead of keeping flexible arteries soft, it can promote inflammation in stiff arteries or destabilize that old plaque, actually *increasing* her risk of a stroke or heart attack.

This is why the strategy changes.

Systemic HRT (Pills/Patches): Generally unsafe to *start* if greater than 10 years since menopause onset. Your doctor may be more or less conservative based on your cardiovascular risk factors.

Local Estrogen (Creams/Tabs): Highly safe and recommended. Local vaginal estrogen doesn't go through the whole system, but it prevents the common urinary tract infections (UTIs) that cause delirium.

Medicine is all about timing. What is a "Longevity Tool" for you at 55 can be a risk for her at 84. This is why we don't treat Barbara like a "smaller, older 55-year-old." She has a narrowed homeostenosis, the rules of maintenance have changed.

🐾 Professor's Facts! 🐾

You might look at Sirius and Leo and wonder if dogs and cats are having hot flashes too.

Surprisingly, no. Domestic animals like dogs and cats do not go through menopause. While their fertility declines with age, they do not experience the sudden, programmed plummet of hormones that human women do.

Humans (and Killer Whales!) are biologically unique in having a long "post-reproductive" life. This means your 55-year-old body is doing something remarkably difficult that even Sirius or Leo doesn't have to contend with. Give yourself some grace. You are navigating a uniquely human biological storm.

Function Over Numbers

We have taken an exhaustive tour of Barbara's classic-model body. This brings us to the most important philosophical shift you must make. In mainstream medicine for younger adults, the focus is often on achieving "perfect numbers": a blood pressure of 120/80, an LDL cholesterol below 100, an A1c below 6.0.

In geriatrics, this focus can be dangerously misguided.

The new goal, the philosophy that should guide every decision you make with Barbara's healthcare team, is **Function Over Numbers**.

The critical question is no longer, "Is the blood pressure 120/80?" The question is, "If we add another medication to get her blood pressure from a perfectly acceptable 140/85 down to 120/80, does that new pill make her so dizzy that she is terrified to walk outside, thus worsening her sarcopenia and isolating her from her friends?" If the pursuit of a "perfect" number destroys her ability to function and enjoy her life, then we have failed, no matter what the lab report says.

The goal of medicine for Barbara is not just to extend her lifespan; it is to maximize her *healthspan* within that life. It is to ensure her remaining years are lived with the highest possible quality of life, with dignity, comfort, and joy. It is to ensure she has the strength to get out of her chair, the balance to walk to the kitchen, and the clarity to enjoy a conversation. That is function. That is our unifying philosophy.

Conclusion: The Master's Touch

Understanding Barbara's body is an act of profound empowerment.

You now understand *why* a small illness creates such discord.

You understand *why* her kidneys require lower doses.

You understand *why* Function, not Numbers, is the goal.

This knowledge illuminates the choice standing before you at your own fifty-five-year-old crossroads. The stiffness, the slowing metabolism—these are the same processes, just in the opening movement.

Our pet companions are the world's greatest professors of observation. Leo cannot tell you his kidney hurts; he tells you by drinking more water. Sirius cannot tell you his hip is stiff; he tells you by hesitating before he climbs the stairs. To care for them, you have had to learn a new language—a language of subtle shifts in behavior, routine, and posture. This skill—the ability to "listen with your eyes"—is the exact same skill required to care for an aging parent whose ability to communicate is changing. Your pets have been preparing you for this role for years.

To navigate this journey for both of you, we need a special set of tools. And as you're about to discover in our next chapter, the most delightful and surprising of these tools are currently curled up asleep in your living room.

It's time to see what your pets can teach you.

What Your Cat and Dog Can Teach You About Medicine, Safety, and Love

If you have ever attempted to give a pill to a cat, you have my deepest and most sincere respect—and I hope you had enough bandages. You have already engaged in a battle of wits, dexterity, and warfare that prepares you for almost any care challenge that lies ahead. That cat, in his defiant, Houdini-like refusal to swallow a gosh-darn tablet, is your first professor of physiology, teaching you about strength, leverage, and the sheer force of will.

Today, we're going to get to know your two resident professors, Leo the cat and Sirius the dog, on a much deeper level. This is a fun detour from the serious business of caring for your aging mother, Barbara, and navigating your own fifty-five-year-old body, but there are lessons to be learned from our loving pets. This chapter, which explores the fascinating details of your pets' biology, is an important part of this book. The lessons learned will guide your transformation from an overwhelmed care partner into a confident, informed advocate for your mother. But before we begin our tour, let's establish the foundational rule that governs all our decisions.

The Guiding Philosophy of This Book

This is not an anti-medication book. To be anti-medication would be to deny the modern miracles that have doubled our lifespan in the last century. The medications in Barbara's pillbox are the result of brilliant science; they prevent strokes, control infections, and allow people with chronic illness to live full, productive lives. With the better blood pressure medications that came around in the 1980s, the rate of strokes has halved. They are critical tools when used with care.

Our goal throughout this book is therefore not to throw away all medications. The goal is to embrace what I call the **"Principle of Less is More"** of medication use. It is a principle of simplicity, elegant precision, of finding just what's needed, nothing more, nothing less, the "just right" spot on the therapeutic spectrum. It is a principle where, before we reach for the next pill, we ask: is the symptom we are trying to solve actually being caused by something else? It's the wisdom that we can overwhelm the body. We don't have to achieve the maximum results, the perfect numbers, if it will detrimentally affect your parent's quality of life. The goal is always to use the right drug, for the right reason, at the lowest effective dose, for the shortest necessary time. Sometimes the right number of drugs is less.

This principle—simplicity, not too many, not too much, but *just right*—is the Guiding Philosophy of responsible geriatric care. It applies to Barbara and her complex needs. It applies to you as you face your own health choices. And as we're about to see, it is a lesson taught most powerfully by the wonderfully different biological systems of your pets.

The Comparative Anatomy Tour

Let's take a guided tour of three distinct, magnificently designed biological machines: your cat Leo, the obligate carnivore; your dog Sirius, the adapted omnivore; and you, the complex, slow-burning omnivore. Their similarities will surprise you, but it is their differences that will teach you the most.

The Digestive Systems: The Specialized to Generalized Gut

The gut is the gateway where the outside world becomes fuel. The profound differences in how these three mammals are engineered to process food tell us almost everything we need to know about their different health risks and needs.

When you look inside Leo, you find the machinery of a pure predator. His entire gastrointestinal (GI) tract is remarkably short—only about three times the length of his body—and it is designed for one purpose: the rapid and efficient digestion of a high-protein, high-fat diet. His stomach is a cauldron of highly concentrated acid, capable of breaking down flesh and neutralizing bacteria. His teeth are tiny daggers for shearing meat, not for grinding plants. His gut is, relative to body length, about half the length of yours. It's a straight, no-nonsense express track, designed to extract nutrients from animal tissue and get waste out *fast*.

Leo's system is a testament to perfect evolutionary design for a specific niche. But this specialization is also a vulnerability. Feeding him a high-carbohydrate diet puts immense strain on a system not designed to handle it. This is a powerful metaphor for elder care. Consider Barbara's eighty-four-year-old digestive system, with its slower motility and reduced enzyme production. It can no longer handle the same foods or medications as your fifty-five-year-old "generalist" system can. Barbara's system has changed enough that we should consider it "specialized;" treating it like a generalist will put tremendous strain on her gut.

As a domesticated descendant of wolves, Sirius represents a beautiful compromise. His GI tract is longer than Leo's but still significantly shorter than yours. His back molars have developed grinding surfaces, showing an adaptation to a more omnivorous diet as a scavenger who could survive on a wider variety of foods [1]. His gut has adapted to live and eat beside us. His system can derive nutrients from both animal and plant sources, but it's still fundamentally geared for a protein-forward diet.

Sirius's cheerful willingness to eat anything you drop is adorable, if not annoying, but it isn't a sign of an invincible gut. In the wild, wolves (Sirius's ancestors) are "gorge and fast" eaters. They evolved to eat massive amounts of meat at once and then go days without food. This is why Sirius will happily eat until he is sick—he has no "off switch" because nature never guaranteed him a next meal. Just because he *wants* it doesn't mean his body *needs* it.

Veterinary clinics see this lesson every day when a dog is rushed in with painful pancreatitis after a dinner of fatty human food or is made ill from eating something astray on the floor or table. He reminds us that just because a system is adaptable, it doesn't mean it's unbreakable. This is a critical lesson for you, the fifty-five-year-old reader. Your body may feel adaptable now, but continually pushing its limits will eventually lead to system failure. Adaptability is not a license for neglect.

The Liver: Three Different Chemical Factories

The liver is the body's magnificent chemical factory, metabolizing nutrients, detoxifying poisons, and processing nearly every medication we ingest. Here, the differences can be a matter of life and death.

Cats are profoundly deficient in a family of liver enzymes called uridine 5'-diphospho-glucuronosyltransferase, or UGTs. This is a mouthful, so let's call it by its function: glucuronidation. This enzyme pathway is one of the body's primary ways of taking a foreign chemical (like a drug), making it water-soluble, and preparing it for elimination [2]. Because of Leo's hyper-carnivorous evolutionary path, where he was seldom exposed to the plant-based toxins many other mammals ate, his liver simply shed the need for this entire pathway.

Imagine his liver has become a specialized chemical processing plant. It does one thing—metabolize proteins and fats—exquisitely and that's what it expects. But if you ask it to process a chemical it is not expecting, the wrong chemical reactions could occur. Because Leo's liver is missing the enzyme for glucuronidation, processing acetaminophen (Tylenol) results in toxic byproducts. These toxic byproducts rapidly build up and destroy the cat's red blood cells and liver tissue. This is why even a tiny fraction of a Tylenol tablet is fatally toxic to a cat.

On the outside, Leo is a perfectly healthy mammal just like

Sirius and us. Internally, the way he processes chemicals is different, sometimes devastatingly so. The same is true of Barbara. Her liver is smaller and has less capacity, and we would be wise to not overwhelm the system. We must be selective, choose the chemicals her liver can handle, and of course, start low and go slow.

Your liver and Sirius's are more versatile. You both have a functional glucuronidation pathway, which is why Tylenol, in the correct dose, is not toxic. However, your factories are still different. A dog's liver often metabolizes certain drugs faster than a human liver.

Similar is not the same. It's tempting to think of a dog as a small person in a fur coat. This is a dangerous assumption. The common human NSAID ibuprofen (Advil) is highly toxic to dogs, causing severe stomach ulcers and kidney failure because their specific metabolic pathways cannot handle it safely [3]. You cannot extrapolate from one individual to another without enormous risk. A medication safe for you is not necessarily safe for your eighty-four-year-old mother. Her internal factory now has its own unique capabilities.

The Kidneys: Three Different Water Management Systems

After the liver processes chemicals, it is the kidneys' job to filter them out of the blood. Evolution has sculpted three remarkably different systems.

Leo's kidneys are a masterpiece of biological engineering. As descendants of desert-dwelling felines, his kidneys are unbelievably efficient at concentrating urine, wringing out and reabsorbing every last drop of water [4]. Cats can concentrate urine two and a half times what we can do, yet their kidneys have only a fifth of the nephrons; this means that cats' kidneys are doing more with less. Hard to look at cleaning the litter box the same way; imagine how much more work it could be.

This high-octane efficiency is also Leo's Achilles' heel. Imagine running an engine constantly at its redline. Over a lifetime, this incredible filtration pressure puts immense strain on his nephrons. Relatively small injuries to a cat's kidneys can result in large reductions in function. It is a major reason why chronic kidney disease (CKD) is an epidemic in older cats. The system designed for his survival in one environment becomes a vulnerability in a long domestic life.

Leo's kidneys teach a powerful lesson about how any system working at peak capacity for years can wear out. It is a direct and poignant parallel to the relentless stress placed on a care partner's own system. Year after year of being "on call" and managing crises can lead to your own burnout. Leo reminds us that even the most efficient systems need rest and support.

Your kidneys and Sirius's are designed for an environment where water is readily available. Their design assumes a regular intake of fluids. Constant dehydration can put immense stress on your kidneys.

Know your operating system's needs. Our kidneys depend on adequate hydration. This becomes critically important for Barbara. The sense of thirst diminishes dramatically in old age leaving many in a constant state of dehydration. A care partner's task, therefore, is ensuring she gets enough fluids to protect her kidneys—a lesson we learn from the fundamental design of our own species' water needs.

Our Parallel Paths of Aging

Aging is universal. The fur around Sirius's muzzle, once a golden blonde, is now a silver-grey. Your once-sleek black cat, Leo, now has his own silver threads. These outward signs mirror the internal changes they share with the humans in your house. Watching them age teaches us what to expect, how to care for Barbara, and how to prepare ourselves.

Joints & Mobility: A Story of Shared Aches

Just like humans, your pets develop osteoarthritis as they age. But they can't tell you their hips hurt. You must become an expert observer. You notice it in your stoic cat, Leo, as a subtle hesitation before he jumps onto the sofa. In Sirius, it's more obvious—the stiffness after a nap, the lagging behind on walks.

The veterinary approach to this problem is a wonderful model for human care. They rarely jump to powerful drugs. The first steps are about function and support:

Orthopedic beds, non-slip rugs, ramps for the car.

Starting with joint supplements like glucosamine, chondroitin, and omega-3 fatty acids [5].

Only if the pain still affects their quality of life do they move to medication, starting with the safest, pet-specific NSAIDs at the lowest effective dose. Never use a human NSAID for a pet, they have their own special needs.

This is a perfect roadmap for Barbara's arthritis. Instead of a new painkiller being the first solution, we should first ask: Are her chairs easy to get out of? Does she have grab bars? Can we try gentle exercise? Sirius's ramp is Barbara's grab bar; both improve function, it just requires some planning and maintenance. The lesson is universal: **Support the function to improve the quality of life.**

Cognition & The Brain

One of the most instructive parallels is the emergence of Canine Cognitive Dysfunction (CCD), or "Doggie Dementia." It's a real, progressive, neurological condition with symptoms that will sound hauntingly familiar: disorientation (getting stuck in corners), changes in social interaction, a disrupted sleep-wake cycle, and loss of learned behaviors [6]. Less is known about the feline experience, but researchers are increasingly recognizing similar signs of cognitive decline in senior cats: howling at night, spatial disorientation, or changes in litter box habits.

Discussing CCD is a powerful, non-threatening way to destigmatize the early signs of human cognitive decline. This is not unique to anyone and there is no shame in it. Seeing these behaviors in a beloved pet frames them not as a personal failure, but as a biological process that requires compassionate management. The strategies we use to help a dog with CCD are precisely the strategies we learn for dementia care:

Predictable routines and schedules reduce anxiety.

A less cluttered space is easier to navigate.

We don't get angry when a dog with CCD has an accident; we calmly clean it up and adjust. This is a visceral lesson in compassionate management.

Lessons in the Principles of Good Care

Leo and Sirius have lots to teach us about the principles of good care.

Keen Observation (The "Leo Framework"). In a system that relies on 8-minute doctor appointments, *you* are the primary diagnostic tool. The system treats what it sees in a snapshot; you treat what you see in the whole photo album of daily life. Your ability to notice a subtle change in appetite or a hesitation on the stairs is more valuable than a once-a-year MRI.

Treat the Patient, Not the Numbers (Function over Numbers). We do not treat lab values; we treat people. A blood pressure of 120/80 is meaningless if the medication required to achieve it makes your mother so dizzy she cannot walk to the mailbox. If a "perfect" number destroys her ability to function, we have failed. Our goal is independence, not data perfection.

Ensuring Safety. Safety is the floor upon which all other care is built. We cannot focus on enrichment or joy if the environment is a minefield of fall risks and medication errors.

Providing Comfort. When cure is no longer possible, comfort becomes the highest form of medicine. We prioritize treatments that relieve suffering over treatments that merely prolong a biological process.

Conclusion: Bringing the Professors' Lessons Home

We have learned some fascinating differences and profound similarities between us and our pets. We now have a newfound appreciation for the unique, intricate biological systems that fill your home, and a set of powerful new principles for care partnerships.

Your pets have taught you the lessons to embrace the

Principle of Less is More of medication use. Leo taught you that on the inside, our bodies are geared towards different needs and functions; his finicky taste for food is his wisdom to avoid what his body cannot handle. Sirius taught you that preserving function without reaching for a medication is a reasonable first approach, and that the precise use of the appropriate medication—when needed—is wise.

With these lessons, you are no longer just an accidental caregiver. You are becoming an informed, compassionate, and confident advocate for everyone in your full house, on two legs and four. Armed with this new perspective, it's time to delve into the modern healthcare system itself and understand the new role you are being asked to play within it.

Navigating the New System

Crossing the threshold from being a supportive child to a medical care partner often feels like entering a foreign country without a map. One day, you are enjoying family dinners and casual phone calls; the next, you are standing under the fluorescent hum of a hospital corridor or staring at a confusing insurance denial letter. You have entered The System.

If you feel overwhelmed, invisible, or like you're constantly shouting into a void, it isn't because you aren't doing enough. The disorientation you feel is a natural response to a fundamental shift in how medicine is practiced today. We are biologically wired to expect a comforting response to illness— assuming that if a member of our community is hurting, the system will intuitively circle the wagons. We expect the doctor to have the time to reflect, the pharmacist to have the bandwidth to double-check every detail, and the hospital to be a quiet sanctuary for healing.

The frustration arises because we are often using old maps in a territory that has fundamentally changed. Over the last few decades, the healthcare infrastructure has transitioned from a localized, slow-paced service model into a highly specialized, fast-paced engine. It works absolute miracles for acute crises—like fixing a broken hip or curing a sudden infection—but it lacks the "connective tissue" required to manage a complex, aging life like Barbara's.

What is missing in this high-speed environment is a **Conductor**.

Because physician specialists often work in separate, soundproof rooms, focusing only on their specific organ or procedure, the overarching coordination that used to hold a medical plan together has largely disappeared.

This is where your advocacy becomes the essential bridge. You are the only one who sees the whole picture of your parent's life, while the system only sees disjointed snapshots. You aren't being difficult when you ask questions or slow things down; you are providing the critical clinical oversight that the system has automated away in exchange for efficiency. And as we will soon see, the confidence required to do this is something you likely already practice every time you take your dog or cat to the veterinarian.

In the coming chapters, we are going to give you the specific tools—the legal "keys," the communication strategies, and the medical frameworks—you need to navigate this new landscape with confidence. You are moving from being a bewildered tourist to becoming a native guide.

The Vet Comparison

Consider what happens when Sirius, the ever-optimistic dog, goes in for his annual checkup. The veterinarian doesn't just quickly listen to his heart and rush out the door. She literally gets down on the floor with him. She hands out yummy treats to win his trust. She asks detailed, probing questions: *"How is his appetite? Is he drinking more water than usual? Does he seem stiff when he gets up in the morning?"* Or think about taking Leo the cat to the clinic.

Leo experiences the world through microscopic movements and ultrasonic hearing, making the chaotic clinic terrifying for him. A good vet knows this. She dims the lights to protect his highly sensitive eyes, speaks in low, soothing tones, and lets him stay in the bottom half of his carrier while she examines him.

The vet looks at the whole animal, their environment, and their daily routine. And most importantly, because Sirius and Leo cannot speak, the veterinarian relies entirely on *you* to tell the story. You are the undisputed expert on their baseline health.

Now, contrast that with taking your eighty-four-year-old mother, Barbara, to her primary care physician. You sit in a sterile room. The doctor comes in, types furiously on a laptop, addresses one specific physical complaint, and is halfway out the door in under ten minutes. It feels disjointed. It feels rushed.

It is easy to walk out of that human clinic feeling frustrated, wondering why your mother's doctor can't be more like Sirius's doctor. Does the vet just care more?

Not at all. The difference isn't a lack of empathy; it is a profound difference in how the two medical systems are built, funded, and operated. To navigate Barbara's care safely and confidently, you don't need to fight the modern medical system, but you do need to understand the unique pressures her human doctors and pharmacists are facing.

The Physician: The 8-minute appointment

Veterinary medicine largely operates on a direct, fee-for-service model. When the vet spends twenty-five minutes examining Sirius and talking to you, that time is built directly into the exam fee. The clinic has the luxury of time because they do not have to negotiate with a third-party insurance company to justify those twenty-five minutes.

Human medicine, however, is tethered to complex insurance networks (like Medicare) that reimburse clinics based on a metric called the RVU (Relative Value Unit). The current RVU system heavily rewards "doing"—like ordering an X-ray, giving an injection, or performing a procedure. Let me be clear, they are not paid for the time they are seeing you, they are paid for the tests they order.

It places a much lower financial value on "thinking"—like spending thirty minutes reviewing a complex, tangled medication history or listening to a patient's fears about memory loss [1].

Consequently, the "8-to-15-minute appointment" is not a choice the doctor is making because they are indifferent; it is a structural reality required to keep the clinic's doors open. This tight schedule makes it incredibly difficult for a physician to notice the subtle, daily signs of decline that you see clearly at home. Furthermore, the human medical system is built on the assumption that adult patients can reliably report their own symptoms. When an older adult begins to experience cognitive decline, that assumption completely breaks down. Just like at the vet, your voice in the exam room becomes the critical bridge between what the doctor sees and what the patient is actually experiencing.

The Pharmacist: The High-Volume Safety Net

Walk into almost any large, modern pharmacy today, and it probably doesn't feel like a quiet healthcare clinic. It feels loud, bright, and overwhelmingly fast. Behind that counter stands one of the most accessible, highly educated clinical experts in your community: your pharmacist. But there is a massive, invisible wall standing between their extensive medical knowledge and your parent's care, and that wall is measured by the ticking of a clock.

The pharmacist is not simply taking pills out of a large bottle and putting them into a smaller one. They are performing a relentless, high-stakes cognitive juggling act. In any given five-minute window, that single pharmacist is clinically verifying a constant stream of complex prescriptions, answering phone calls from frustrated doctors' offices, untangling insurance rejections, administering vaccines, and managing a backed-up drive-thru window.

The structure of modern retail pharmacy requires them to work at astonishing speeds, sometimes verifying prescriptions in a matter of seconds [2]. Because of the sheer velocity of their day, the pharmacist has to rely heavily on the computer's automated safety alerts. The computer is fantastic at catching obvious, immediate dangers—like an antibiotic that fatally interacts with a blood thinner. But the computer doesn't know what over-the-counter medications your parents are taking unless you let the pharmacy staff know to update their system.

The computer is completely blind to the slow, nuanced reality of an aging body. A computer screen doesn't know that Barbara has lost ten pounds this month that could be a side effect, also meaning a "normal" dose of a medication might now be too strong. Catching these subtle, long-term issues requires a clinician to sit down, look at the whole patient, and think critically.

That pharmacist desperately wants to talk to you. When you step up to the counter and ask for a brief consultation about your mother's medications, you give them the structural permission they need to pause the timer, step away from the chaos, and use their hard-earned expertise to protect your parent. You just have to be the one to raise your hand.

The Hospital: The Focus on Stabilization

We often view hospitals as peaceful sanctuaries for long-term rest and recovery, much like they were in the mid-twentieth century. Today, they are designed to be high-efficiency stabilization centers.

Under the modern Medicare Diagnosis-Related Group (DRG) system, hospitals receive a fixed payment based on the patient's specific diagnosis (like a hip fracture or pneumonia), regardless of how many days the patient stays in the bed [3]. This means their primary, life-saving goal is to stabilize the acute crisis—to stop the bleeding, clear the infection, or fix the bone—and then swiftly transition the patient to a rehabilitation center or home to finish the slow work of healing.

The hospital staff aren't trying to rush Barbara out the door unkindly; they are simply fulfilling their specific role in the medical pipeline, stabilizing her so they can make room for the next acute emergency. It's how efficiency plays out in our modern hospitals.

The Anatomy of a Systems Error: The Triple Whammy
When we have incredibly talented specialists operating in their own fast-paced lanes, we often experience a "Coordination Gap." The cardiologist plays their part for the heart, the nephrologist plays for the kidneys, and the primary care doctor manages the daily aches. But because they are moving so fast, no one is looking at the whole patient.

To understand why your involvement is so necessary, consider a common clinical scenario known as the *Triple Whammy*.

1. It begins when Barbara's primary care doctor prescribes **Lisinopril** for her blood pressure. It is a great, protective medication.
2. A few weeks later, a specialist notices her ankles are swollen and prescribes a diuretic, **Furosemide** (a

"water pill"). This is also a perfectly standard treatment.

3. Unbeknownst to her doctors, Barbara has also started taking over-the-counter **Ibuprofen** every morning for a flare-up of knee pain.

Individually, these three medications make perfect sense. But taken together in an older body, they alter the blood flow in and out of the kidneys in a specific way that can cause the kidneys to suffer acute injury and even shut down [4].

This dangerous interaction is sometimes missed because the doctors' computer systems aren't always linked, the OTC painkiller isn't on the official chart, and the pharmacist does not have the time to ask about those OTCs.

This isn't a failure of the people caring for her; it is a blind spot in a highly specialized system. The system requires a unifying voice to see the whole board. It requires someone to step back, look at the big picture, and say, *"Wait a minute, how do all these separate pieces fit together?"* That person is you.

5 | THE CONDUCTOR

Stepping into Your Empowering New Role

If you reflect on the realities of modern medicine we just explored—the fast-paced clinics, the high-volume pharmacies, the hospital wards built for rapid stabilization—you might notice something missing. The system functions like a sprawling orchestra of incredibly talented musicians. The cardiologist plays a beautiful melody for the heart, the nephrologist plays a complex rhythm for the kidneys, and the pharmacist expertly tunes the instruments.

But because they are all playing in separate rooms, moving at breakneck speed, there is no one standing on the conductor's podium. The system is no longer designed to provide a central coordinator. That seat is currently empty.

This is not a cause for despair; it is a profound opportunity. As Barbara's care partner, you are the only person in her life perfectly positioned to step onto that podium. You do not need to be a *musician*—you don't need to know how to perform surgery or memorize complex pharmacology. Your job as the Conductor is simply to ensure all the talented specialists are looking at the exact same sheet of music.

The Skills You Already Have: Lessons from Sirius and Leo

Taking on the role of Conductor can sound intimidating, but I promise you already have the exact skill set required to do it beautifully. To prove it, let's look back at Sirius and Leo.

When Sirius the dog gets a new chewable joint supplement and suddenly stops eating his dinner, you don't wait six months for his next annual vet appointment to figure out what went wrong. You notice the change in his baseline behavior by that very same evening, simply because you are the one filling his bowl.

When Leo the cat is prescribed a specialized diet for his kidneys, you don't just blindly pour the kibble and hope for the best. You actively monitor him. You notice how often he visits the water bowl, you pay attention to how he uses the litter box, and when you take him back to the vet, you deliver a highly detailed report on his daily habits.

You do this effortlessly because you recognize that you are their Chief Medical Officer. You know that the vet only sees a ten-minute snapshot of their lives, while you see the entire album.

Stepping into the role of the Conductor for your aging parent requires this exact same observational mindset. You don't need a medical degree to know that Barbara is suddenly struggling to balance when she stands up, or that she seems unusually confused after taking her new bladder medication. You just have to trust your daily observations and be willing to share your observation with her doctors.

Why You Are the Perfect Leader

You are uniquely qualified to fill this role for three very specific reasons:

1. The medical computer only knows what is officially typed into it. It doesn't know that Barbara skips her afternoon pill because it upsets her stomach, or that she takes an over-the-counter sleep aid every night that isn't on the official chart. You hold the missing pieces of the puzzle that her doctors desperately need to make safe decisions.

2. Every professional in the healthcare system is balancing the needs of a packed waiting room, a busy pharmacy queue, or a hospital floor. You are the only person in the room whose sole, undivided focus is Barbara's actual quality of life and functional independence.

3. In a medical system built for speed, your calm, prepared presence serves as the necessary pause button. By asking the right questions, you help the machinery slow down and acknowledge your mother as a whole, complex person rather than just a quick appointment slot.

Taking on this role does not mean you are being difficult or demanding. In fact, you are providing the essential coordination that rushed doctors and pharmacists desperately need for them to do their best work.

The Price of Admission: The Legal Keys

There is, however, one major difference between managing Leo's care and managing Barbara's care. When you take a cat to the vet, you are legally recognized as the owner, so the vet can tell you anything. Human healthcare is entirely different. It is bound by strict, federal privacy laws designed to protect the patient.

Before you can step onto the podium and act as the

Conductor, you must secure the legal authority to do so. Think of these documents as your "Price of Admission." Without them, the system's doors will remain firmly locked, no matter how much you want to help [1].

To transform from a supportive visitor into the recognized voice of the patient, you need to work with your parent to get these four specific tools into your toolkit:

- **The HIPAA Release:** This is the communication key. Without a signed HIPAA (Health Insurance Portability and Accountability Act) release on file at the doctor's office and the pharmacy, the medical staff cannot legally discuss medications, test results, or upcoming appointments with you. Getting this signed while your parent is still cognitively healthy is step one.

- **Medical Power of Attorney (MPOA):** This is the decision-making key. Also known as a healthcare proxy, this document legally designates you as the person who will make medical decisions if your parent becomes unable to speak for themselves (due to dementia, a stroke, or severe illness). Without an MPOA, the medical system must legally default to its automatic settings—which almost always means doing "more" interventions, even if that isn't what your parent would have wanted.

- **Financial Power of Attorney:** This is the logistical key. Medical care is deeply intertwined with finances. If your parent needs to transition to a memory care facility or requires in-home nursing, you need the legal authority to access their bank accounts to pay for that care.

- **POLST or Living Will:** A POLST (Physician Orders for Life-Sustaining Treatment) is the emergency key. This is a brightly colored medical order that sits on the patient's refrigerator. It tells paramedics and ER staff exactly what your parent's wishes are regarding CPR, ventilators, and feeding tubes. In a crisis, paramedics are trained to act fast and keep the patient alive at all costs. A POLST ensures they pause and respect your parent's specific boundaries [2].

Having these keys in your hands ensures that when a crisis hits, you don't have to waste precious time arguing with hospital administrators about whether you have the right to speak up. You are already officially on the record.

Tools of the Trade

So, what does it actually look like when the Conductor steps up with their legal keys in hand? Let's revisit the dangerous *Triple Whammy* scenario from the previous chapter—where the combination of blood pressure pills, water pills, and over-the-counter pain relievers threatened to shut down Barbara's kidneys.

When a Conductor is present, that danger is entirely avoided through simple, highly effective tools that we will learn in this book.

First, when Barbara develops knee pain, you don't just show up to the doctor's office and hope the physician remembers her kidney function. You arrive with a **One-Page Briefing**. This is a simple piece of paper you hand to the doctor at the very beginning of the eight-minute appointment. It lists her current medications (including that over-the-counter ibuprofen) and states your primary goal: *"Goal today: Treat knee pain safely alongside her current blood pressure regimen."* Second, you also bring your updated **Medication List**. Because you provided this clear, synthesized data, you save the doctor time. The doctor immediately sees the risk, skips the pills, and prescribes a safe topical pain gel instead.

Third, if she does need a new prescription down the road, you utilize the **Brown Bag Consult**—a well-known tool of pharmacists. You take all her pill bottles—prescriptions, vitamins, and supplements—put them in a literal brown bag, and take them to your local pharmacist [3]. You ask for a brief, dedicated consultation to review how the new drug fits with the old ones. This gives the pharmacist the moment they need to step out of the fast-paced retail workflow, review the whole picture, and catch any hidden interactions that a fragmented computer system might have missed.

The One-Page Briefing, Medication List, and Brown Bag Consult are just a few tools you will learn in this book. You will also learn how to navigate the ER, hospitalizations, and how to audit a nursing home if that becomes necessary. By the end of this book, you will have all the tools you need to be the master Conductor of your parent's medical care. You'll have the tools for all the medical specialists to make beautiful music together.

The patient is the same, the symptoms are the same, and the medical professionals remain the same. By acting as the Conductor, you ensure Barbara stays safe, healthy, and independent in her own home.

Stepping into the role of the Conductor is a fundamental shift from being an anxious bystander to becoming a confident leader of your parent's health. You are no longer just a concerned child navigating a confusing system; you are a savvy partner equipped with a master strategy. You are the Conductor. And it is time to make some beautiful coordinated music.

PART 3 | THE FLIP

From the *Path to the Pillbox*... to the *Path of Fewer Pills, More Paws*

For the first half of this book, we have learned that the *Path to the Pillbox* is the default path. You can continue down the same path as Barbara with little effort; this is where we are all headed.

But now, we are going to flip the script.

We have to acknowledge a hard truth: Barbara didn't choose the *Path to the Pillbox*. She ended up there because, for most of her life, it was the only path available. The science of longevity and neuroplasticity was in its infancy. Doctors didn't know about the "Glymphatic System" or "Metabolic Reserve." They didn't have the data we have now. They did the best they could with the tools they had, which mostly meant treating every new symptom with a new prescription.

But in the last decade, the lights have been turned on. Landmark clinical trials like the FINGER and U.S. POINTER studies have finally given us the data we were missing. We now know—with scientific certainty—what actually keeps the mind sharp and the body resilient.

Barbara didn't have this map. **You do.**

This section is "The Flip." We are flipping from defense to

offense. We are flipping from treating the number to treating the person. And we are flipping the trajectory of your own aging process so that twenty years from now, you won't be standing in the pharmacy line.

Interrupting the Path to the Pillbox

You start your day, as always, in a rush. The alarm feels like an assault. You skip a real breakfast in favor of a coffee that you drink while answering overnight work emails and mentally preparing for the day's first meeting. You fold the laundry you didn't get to finish last night, notice a passive-aggressive text from a sibling about your mother's care, and realize you forgot to take the chicken out of the freezer for dinner. As you finally grab your keys, your heart is pounding with a familiar, low-grade thrum of anxiety. You pause, take a breath, and tell yourself this is just the price of a busy, modern life. It's normal.

On the drive to work, you take a handful of ibuprofen for the ache in your lower back that has become your constant companion. Later that day, you'll fight off the 3 p.m. slump with another coffee and a sugary snack from the vending machine. Dinner will be something quick and processed. You'll collapse onto the couch, intending to watch one show, but will end up scrolling on your phone for two hours, your mind too tired to sleep but too wired to rest. When you finally get into bed, your brain whirs with your endless to-do list.

This is the portrait of a competent, caring, and completely overwhelmed fifty-five-year-old. This is, for so many of us, normal.

This chapter is about connecting the dots. It is about drawing a straight, undeniable line from this "normal" day to the crowded, rainbow-colored pill organizer that sits on your mother's nightstand—and is quietly waiting to take up residence on your own.

The *Path to the Pillbox* does not begin with a catastrophic illness. It doesn't start with a heart attack or a stroke. It begins silently, almost invisibly, with the first "harmless" pill prescribed to treat the predictable downstream effect of a life lived on the brink of burnout. This chapter is a cautionary tale, but it is not about blame or fear. It is about illumination. By understanding the anatomy of this common and preventable cascade, you gain the power to choose a different destination.

The First Domino: The "Harmless" Blood Pressure Pill

The tipping point begins not in a hospital, but in the familiar, sterile environment of your primary care doctor's office during your annual physical. You are fifty-five. You feel... fine. Tired, yes. Stressed, absolutely. But not sick.

The medical assistant wraps the cuff around your arm. It tightens, then slowly releases. The doctor comes in, reviews your chart, and says the words that so many millions of people in your exact position have heard: *"Well, your blood pressure is a little elevated today. It's 145/90. We'll check it again before you leave, but this is the third time it's been high. Let's start you on something. It's a very low dose of a water pill, a thiazide diuretic like hydrochlorothiazide. It's extremely common, very safe, and it should bring this right down."*

You agree, because it seems like the responsible thing to do.

High blood pressure is serious, and the solution seems so simple. You pick up the prescription, a small white pill you now take every morning. You feel a sense of relief. Problem solved.

But what *really* happened? You have just placed the first domino in a long, wobbly line. The pill is not the problem; the pill is an elegant biochemical solution to a pressure problem. The real issue is the decade of physiological changes we discussed in Chapter 1 that led to this moment: the slow, age-related stiffening of your arteries, the gradual loss of muscle mass (sarcopenia), and the chronic, low-grade stress elevating your cortisol and constricting your blood vessels. In an 8-minute appointment, writing a prescription is the most efficient way to close the encounter. The system is built for speed, not for 30-minute lifestyle conversations.

The little white pill does its job beautifully. It makes your kidneys flush out more salt and water, reducing the fluid volume in your stiff "garden hose," and your blood pressure comes down. On paper, you are now healthier. But this is where our story truly begins, because every action in pharmacology has a reaction. And all too often, the consequences of the first pill are treated with a second.

The Domino Effect: An Introduction to the Prescribing Cascade

Before we follow our first domino, I need to introduce you to one of the most important concepts in geriatric medicine: the **Prescribing Cascade**.

As first described by Drs. Rochon and Gurwitz [1], a prescribing cascade occurs when an adverse drug event—a side effect—is misinterpreted as a new medical condition, leading to the prescription of a second, potentially unnecessary medication to treat that side effect.

Let that sink in.

Pill #1 is prescribed for Condition A.

Pill #1 causes a side effect.

That side effect is not recognized as being drug-related. Instead, it is diagnosed as new Condition B.

Pill #2 is prescribed to treat Condition B.

This cycle can continue, adding more pills, more side effects, more risk, and more complexity, until a person is trapped in a web of treatments for conditions that were actually caused by their initial treatments. It is a quiet epidemic hiding in plain sight.

The Second Domino: A "New" Bladder Problem

You've been on your hydrochlorothiazide (HCTZ) for six months. Your blood pressure is better. But you've noticed a new and troubling problem. You have to pee. *All the time.*

You find yourself mapping out every public restroom. Long car rides require strategic planning. You're waking up two or three times a night, disrupting your already fragile sleep. So, you go back to your doctor. You describe your symptoms: *"Doctor, I have this incredible urgency to urinate, and I'm going so frequently. It's really affecting my quality of life."*

You might not think to mention the blood pressure pill you started half a year ago. It seems unrelated, after all you're getting older. The doctor, hearing your symptoms, does exactly what their training has prepared them to do. They recognize a classic clinical picture. "It sounds like you've developed an overactive bladder, or OAB," they might say. "It's very common as people age. Don't worry, we have a medication for that."

You have just been diagnosed with a new medical condition. But is it one? The scientific literature provides a clear answer. Multiple studies have shown a significant link between diuretic use and urinary incontinence symptoms. For instance, a large 2016 study found that older adults taking diuretics were **more than twice as likely** to suffer from urinary urgency—that desperate, "I have to go *right now*" feeling [2]. Your 'new' condition isn't new at all; it is a direct, predictable side effect of your first pill.

But because the symptom so perfectly mimics the diagnosis of Overactive Bladder, the dots were not connected. And so, you leave the pharmacy with **Pill #2**: a medication for overactive bladder, very likely an anticholinergic drug like oxybutynin (Ditropan) or tolterodine (Detrol). You have taken a step down the prescribing cascade.

The Third Domino: The Onset of Brain Fog

Your new bladder medication works. The constant urgency subsides. But over the next few months, a different, more insidious symptom emerges. It's that feeling we identified earlier, The Overloaded Brain, but amplified. The "brain fog" is thicker. Words seem to be just out of reach more often. You feel a persistent, unpleasant dryness in your mouth. You're also becoming more constipated.

You become increasingly worried. This cognitive slowing is deeply frightening. What is happening? You have just run headfirst into the profound and often-underappreciated side effects of **anticholinergic** drugs.

Acetylcholine is a master neurotransmitter in your brain, essential for learning, memory formation, and concentration. Bladder medications like oxybutynin work by blocking acetylcholine's action, but they do so not just in the bladder but also cross the blood-brain barrier, directly undermining the very neurochemical processes you need to think clearly [3]. The dry mouth and constipation are also classic anticholinergic side effects.

The link between a high "anticholinergic burden" and cognitive impairment is a scientific fact. A landmark 2015 study in *JAMA Internal Medicine*, following nearly 3,500 people, found a stunning dose-response relationship: the higher the anticholinergic dose and the longer the use, the greater the risk of developing dementia [4]. A subsequent study in 2018 confirmed this, showing that the highest exposure to these drugs was associated with an almost **50% increased risk of dementia** [5].

You are, in a very real sense, taking a pill that is dulling your mind to treat a side effect of a pill that is lowering your blood pressure. This is the prescribing cascade in its most dangerous form. Remember the Triple Whammy scenario in Chapter 4? That was a Prescribing Cascade. Now, we are going to look at the mechanics of how to stop it before it starts.

Rewinding the Tape: How This Story Could Have Been Different

This cascade feels inevitable, but it is not. At every single step, there were opportunities—off-ramps from the *Path to the Pillbox*—that you could have taken. The power lies in knowing where they are.

> ### 🔑 Pharmacist Pro Tip! 🔑
>
> If you see the letters **"PM"** on a box (Tylenol PM, Advil PM), put it back on the shelf. The "PM" ingredient is almost always **Diphenhydramine** (Benadryl). In a 30-year-old, it makes you sleepy. In an 80-year-old, it blocks acetylcholine, the chemical your brain needs to form memories. It is a known trigger for delirium and falls [6]. If Barbara needs sleep, try melatonin or magnesium first—leave the "PM" for the young.

Interruption Point #1: The Initial Diagnosis

The doctor says, *"Your blood pressure is 145/90. Let's start you on a water pill."*

Instead of passively accepting, you engage as a partner. You ask, *"I understand. Before we start a medication I might be on for life, are there any lifestyle approaches we could try first for a few months? I'm willing to work hard on this."*

This is evidence-based medicine. Landmark clinical trials on the DASH (Dietary Approaches to Stop Hypertension) diet have shown it can lower blood pressure as effectively as a single medication [7]. Furthermore, meta-analyses of randomized controlled trials consistently show that a modest weight loss of just 5% of body weight (about 8-10 pounds for many people) can produce a clinically significant reduction in blood pressure [8]. Imagine preventing the entire cascade with a focused, three-month effort on diet and daily walks.

Interruption Point #2: The Bladder Symptoms Appear

You notice the new, urgent need to urinate constantly.

Before assuming it's a new disease, you practice the most important question in medication management: "Could this be a side effect?" You call your pharmacist and say, "*I started hydrochlorothiazide six months ago, and now I have this new urgency. Could the two be related?*" A good pharmacist will immediately confirm the link.

Armed with this information, you can have a different conversation with your doctor. They now have new options:

Lower the dose of the hydrochlorothiazide to see if it lessens the side effect.

Switch to another class of blood pressure medication, like an ACE inhibitor or an ARB, which do not have this diuretic effect.

Encourage physical therapy. This is not a typo. Cochrane reviews, the gold standard for medical evidence, have shown that pelvic floor muscle training is a highly effective first-line treatment for improving urinary urgency and incontinence, directly strengthening the systems that support bladder function without adding another chemical [9].

Interruption Point #3: The Fear of Brain Fog

You're taking the bladder medication, and you feel the onset of brain fog.

Again, you ask: "*Could this be a side effect?*" You are now a seasoned pro at this.

The Science-Backed Alternative: The goal now is to stop the offending anticholinergic drug. But this is also a moment to zoom out and see how interconnected the body is. You are experiencing The Overloaded Brain, amplified by a medication. This is a catalyst to build cognitive resilience.

When you come home, frazzled and worried about your memory, your dog Sirius doesn't offer a pill. He nudges his head into your hand. The simple, rhythmic act of petting him has been shown to lower cortisol and blood pressure. A brisk walk outside with him, focused only on the path ahead and his joyful sniffing, is a powerful form of mindfulness that breaks the cycle of anxious thoughts.

Your cat Leo is a Zen master. He can sit in a sunbeam, utterly present, for an hour. He is not multitasking. He is a model of the focused attention that is the direct antidote to The Overloaded Brain.

This isn't just a quaint idea; it's hard science. Regular physical activity boosts a crucial protein called Brain-Derived Neurotrophic Factor (BDNF), which is like fertilizer for your brain cells, helping them grow and form new connections [10]. Both short-term and long-term exercise have been robustly linked to improved executive function, memory, and processing speed—the very functions that feel compromised when you're experiencing brain fog [11].

Treat the Patient, Not the Numbers

In our world of uncertainty, it might be comforting to see that our vitals and lab numbers are falling in the "good" range. But paying too much attention to "perfect" values can make the prescribing cascade worse. Chasing the "good" blood pressure of 120/80, an A1C below 7.0, and a cholesterol level that fits a guideline seems tempting. We just need to add another pill or increase the dose to fix the number. This might be fine in the 30-year-old body, but the narrow homeostenosis of an 84-year-old has a distinct physiology. To understand why, it might be helpful to see how those perfect numbers are established.

Most of those numbers are established in a sample of healthy 20–40-year-olds, usually male weighing an average of 70 kg (154 pounds). How similar does this sound to Barbara? As we age, what we consider "normal" needs an update.

Instead of treating to the good numbers, treating to a functional range—where Barbara is able to walk, think, and eat without side effect—is far more optimal.

Conclusion: Interrupting the Domino

At every step of this journey, from the first domino to the last, the *Path to Fewer Pills, More Paws* offered an alternative. That alternative wasn't always easy, but it was always empowering. It was a path that asked "why," looked for root causes, and favored simple, powerful, biological solutions over the deceptively simple fix of the next pill. The *Path to the Pillbox* is paved with good intentions and unasked questions. You now know the questions to ask. This is one of the biggest reasons I think a revolution is coming for geriatric care.

7 | The *Path to Fewer Pills, More Paws*

The Strategy

We took a hard, honest look at the *Path to the Pillbox*. We traced the all-too-common route from a "normal," stressed-out life to a medicine cabinet overflowing with amber vials. It was a cautionary tale, drawing a straight line from the chronic stress and sedentary habits of middle age to the physiological frailty of later life.

It reveals the fork in the road. Now, we flip the map over. It is time to chart the course for the alternative route: The *Path to Fewer Pills, More Paws*.

This chapter is your "how-to." It is your practical, actionable guide to building a life that resists polypharmacy. We are not looking for a magical fountain of youth, nor are we interested in adding more impossible tasks to your already overwhelmed to-do list. We are looking for something far more sustainable.

We are looking for the kind of vitality we see every day in our living rooms. Think of Sirius. He doesn't worry about his cholesterol or stress about his 401(k). He simply lives. When he runs for a ball, he is pure kinetic energy. When he rests, he is fully at rest. He and Leo possess an innate biological wisdom that we have lost—a way of living that prioritizes function, nourishment, and recovery. This chapter is about reclaiming that wisdom for ourselves.

Healthspan over Lifespan

To understand this strategy, we must introduce a concept that is the absolute gold standard in modern gerontology: **Healthspan**.

Our goal is specific: Healthspan over Lifespan.

Lifespan is simply the number of years you breathe. It is a statistic on a death certificate. Modern medicine is incredibly good at extending lifespan; we can keep hearts beating and lungs inflating long after the quality of life has vanished. That is the trap of the *Path to the Pillbox*—a long life spent managing decline.

Healthspan is different. Healthspan is the number of those years you *live*—with vitality, a clear mind, and the functional independence to enjoy your time. It is the ability to walk Sirius around the block without pain when you are eighty. It is the clarity of mind to read a book with Leo on your lap without the fog of medication. It is the difference between surviving your final decades and thriving in them.

The High-5 for Healthspan

When I was a professor, students would often come to me during office hours. They would ask, sometimes sheepishly, sometimes not so sheepishly, "Professor... what's going to be on the test?"

They didn't want the fluff. They were busy, stressed, and overwhelmed—much like you are now. They wanted the diamonds of truth in the rough. They wanted to know exactly where to focus their limited energy to get the best result.

Well, I'm going to give you the truths. I am going to give you the strategies you need so you don't have to spend years doing the research yourself. My intention is to give you the highest-yield, most time-efficient, science-backed strategies to maximize your healthspan.

For years, we looked for a single magic pill to prevent cognitive decline. But the landmark FINGER and U.S. POINTER studies have finally given us the answer, and it wasn't a pill at all. These studies proved that the secret lies in a "multidomain" approach. They showed that when you target five distinct biological systems simultaneously, you create a shield that is stronger than the sum of its parts. You cannot ignore one. This multidomain approach is the key.

I call this the **High-5 for Healthspan**. Your health requires all five of these biological systems working in unison. If you ignore one, the system fails. These elements are: **Physical, Nutritional, Vascular, Cognitive & Social, and Restorative Health**.

First Some Good News…Your DNA is Not Your Destiny
Many of us live in fear of the "Alzheimer's Gene," ApoE4. You may have gotten one of those DNA tests and the results give you cold sweats at night and think to yourself, *"This is my inevitable future."*

The science has definitive news for you: **You are not doomed.**

The FINGER and U.S. POINTER studies analyzed this specific fear [1, 2]. They separated participants into those with the high-risk gene (ApoE4 carriers) and those without.

The lifestyle interventions worked **just as well, and potentially even better,** for the people with the high-risk gene [3].

Your genes load the gun, but your lifestyle pulls the trigger. But modest efforts, over time, caring for your body can zero out that risk as if it were not there. If you provide that care—via modest exercise, the MIND diet, and optimizing vascular health—you can override your genetic risk.

1. Physical Health

We begin with the muscles and bones that carry you through the world. If there were a single pill that could lower your blood pressure, manage your insulin, and grow new brain connections, it would be a trillion-dollar drug. That pill doesn't exist but something else can achieve those same results—exercise. Groan, I know! But you don't have to be a marathon runner, just small daily efforts. To fight the two great thieves of aging—**Sarcopenia** (muscle loss) and **Frailty**—we need to be specific. Here are the exercises the clinical studies showed make the difference for cognitive and physical independence. They are achievable through small daily efforts.

Resistance Training: This is the single most important type of exercise for a fifty-five-year-old. As we learned, sarcopenia (the loss of muscle mass) is the silent engine driving so many age-related problems. The only way to stop it is to actively fight it with resistance training.

When you challenge your muscles with a load heavier than what they are used to, it creates tiny tears in the muscle fibers. Your body responds by rebuilding them slightly thicker and stronger. This process improves the efficiency of the nerves that fire your muscles and rebuilds the metabolic "sponges" that soak up blood sugar [4].

You do not need a fancy gym. You need to consistently challenge your major muscle groups two to three times a week for about 20-30 minutes. Begin with bodyweight exercises. A squat (sitting down and standing up from a chair without using your hands) is one of the most functional exercises on earth, strengthening the very muscles you need to stay independent. A push-up (done against a wall or counter) builds upper body strength. As you get stronger, add inexpensive resistance bands or light dumbbells.

Aim to feel a "burn"—the feeling of your muscles working hard—by the end of a set of 8-12 repetitions. That feeling is the signal you are creating the stimulus for growth.

For women especially, resistance training is non-negotiable. Because of the bone density lost during menopause, your skeleton needs the pull of muscle to stay strong.

Weight-bearing exercise isn't just about looking toned; it is the only way to signal your bones to hold onto their mineral density. Every time you lift a weight, the muscle pulls on the bone, and the bone responds by getting tougher. It is your insurance policy against frailty.

Cardiovascular: We've established that our arteries get stiffer with age. Consistent cardiovascular exercise is the best tool we have to improve their health. The most sustainable and beneficial type of cardio for long-term health is Zone 2 training.

Zone 2 refers to a low-to-moderate intensity level, about 60-70% of your maximum heart rate. This is the "conversational" pace—you should be able to hold a conversation, but not sing. Training in this zone is particularly effective at improving mitochondrial efficiency. Mitochondria are the tiny power plants inside your cells. Zone 2 training increases both the number and the efficiency of your mitochondria, turning your body into a more efficient, fat-burning, all-day-energy machine. Zone 2 is what the research aims for, this is where most people get the most benefits and lowest risk of injuries. The key is not to push yourself, be reasonable and honest with your goals. Get the recommendations of a doctor, physical therapist, or occupational therapist.

Aim for 150 minutes per week, broken down however you like. A brisk 30-minute walk with Sirius five days a week. Two 45-minute bike rides. The key is consistency.

Think of Sirius. He doesn't just sit on the porch; he patrols. Movement is his default state. He understands that a body in motion stays in motion, and by adopting his habit of daily patrol, we generate **BDNF** (Brain-Derived Neurotrophic Factor), a protein that acts like fertilizer for our brain cells. Exercise directly supports brain health.

2. Nutritional Health

For years, we've been told to simply "eat healthy." What does that mean? Low fat? No carbs?

For the fifty-five-year-old body, we need to be more specific. We aren't just feeding a body; we are protecting a brain. The FINGER study proved that specific nutrients can reduce inflammation and preserve the brain's wiring.

We combine the need for muscle-building protein with the protective power of the MIND Diet [5]. Add berries and greens to your diet. And, we make friends with fiber and frenemies with "Hyper-Palatable." The sum total is an anti-inflammatory diet.

Prioritize Protein: Protein is the building block of muscle, and fighting sarcopenia is your top priority. Due to the "anabolic resistance" of aging, you need *more* protein than a younger person. Many geriatric experts now recommend 1.2 to 1.6 grams of protein per kilogram of body weight for optimal health [6]. Don't get lost in calculations. Just make sure every meal is centered around a significant source of lean protein—eggs, Greek yogurt, chicken, fish, tofu, or lentils. For most people, this looks like a palm-sized portion of chicken or salmon at lunch and dinner, plus two eggs at breakfast.

Strawberries, Blueberries and Leafy Greens: Spinach, kale, and blueberries are packed with compounds that clear oxidative stress. These specific foods were shown to support brain health because of their anti-inflammatory properties.

Olive oil: We swap butter for olive oil and chips for nuts to provide the high-quality lipids our brain needs to maintain its structure. They are also less inflammatory than saturated fats. Your brain is the fattiest organ in the body—60% of its structural weight is pure fat. This makes your diet a direct supply chain for your brain's hardware. Think about the grease in a bacon pan: when it cools, it turns white, waxy, and hard. Now think about olive oil: it stays golden and fluid. Which material do you want surrounding your delicate neurons? We swap butter for olive oil not to lose weight, but to keep our brain chemistry fluid.

Fiber is Your Friend: The fiber found in vegetables, fruits, and legumes is critical for your metabolic and gut health. It helps lower cholesterol, stabilizes blood sugar, and feeds the beneficial bacteria in your gut—your microbiome—which plays a crucial role in everything from your immune system to your mood [7]. One of my friends calls it "eating the rainbow." Fill half your plate at every meal with colorful, non-starchy vegetables.

Fear the "Hyper-Palatable": The biggest nutritional enemy you face is the modern food industry's mastery of creating "hyper-palatable" processed foods. These are products scientifically engineered with fat, sugar, and salt to be irresistible and bypass your body's satiety signals. The clichés apply: Eat whole, real food. If it came in a crinkly bag with a long list of ingredients you can't pronounce, treat it as an occasional treat.

In this, we look to Leo. You may think of him as finicky, but he is actually discerning. Remember his specialized gut? He refuses to eat "junk." He knows instinctively what is nourishment and what is filler. We must treat our own bodies with the same discernment, avoiding the hyper-palatable processed foods that spike our insulin and starve our brains.

3. Vascular Health

Throughout this book, I've told you not to obsess over numbers. But there is a crucial exception. Your brain is a vascular organ, fed by miles of delicate blood vessels that supply it with oxygen. We must ensure those vessels remain open and flexible.

The SPRINT-MIND trial proved that aggressively managing your blood pressure is the single most effective way to prevent Mild Cognitive Impairment [8]. High pressure creates micro-tears in the delicate vessels of your brain, leading to damage that manifests decades later.

This is the non-negotiable part of the strategy. You must

know your 3 Numbers: your **blood pressure**, your **blood sugar**, and your **cholesterol**. We try to manage these with diet and exercise first. But—and this is critical—if those lifestyle changes do not bring your blood pressure down, *this is the time when a pill is the right answer*. At fifty-five, protecting your brain from the physical damage of pressure is worth the medication. There may be a time when aggressively managing these numbers could be detrimental. At eighty-four, managing function over numbers may very well be the right call.

4. Cognitive & Social Health

We've talked about training the muscles in your legs and arms. But the most vital "muscle" we need to exercise to ensure a long healthspan resides between our ears. Keeping your brain active, challenged, and engaged is not a luxury; it is a fundamental aspect of proactive health.

The goal here is to build **Cognitive Reserve.** This theory posits that individuals who engage in mentally stimulating activities build a denser, more complex, and more efficient network of neural connections. This dense network acts as a powerful buffer against age-related changes. It's like having a vast, interconnected system of roads; if one main highway is closed, there are hundreds of other routes to your destination. It builds resilience and flexibility that would get lost with age.

Your brain is stimulated only when it's being pushed just beyond its comfort zone. The key is finding a complex skill that is so engaging you *want* to stick with it. Remember a core principle here: mastering a complex skill is more enriching, and neurologically beneficial, than the fleeting thrill of a single parachute jump.

Learn a New Language: This engages multiple cognitive systems at once: memory, auditory processing, and executive function.

But we cannot do this alone, we need **Social Engagement**. Social Isolation shrinks the brain. We are social animals, and we wither without the "Pack." We need to connect with other humans or animals every single day. Keep your parent socially engaged. Knitting, bridge, golf, whatever they find fun and engaging.

One lesson from this might be simple: Don't just walk the dog; *train* the dog. Teaching Sirius a new trick is the perfect multidomain exercise. It is physical, it requires cognitive focus, and it is deeply social. That engagement and novelty keep both of your brains young.

5. Restorative Health

For many years, sleep was treated as a luxury. We now know that this view is catastrophically wrong. Sleep is an active, essential biological process that is non-negotiable for health. Stress management is essential to reduce the cortisol bathing your brain. For the fifty-five-year-old battling The Overloaded Brain, it is the single most powerful tool you have.

Sleep: Your brain has a specialized cleaning mechanism called the Glymphatic System, but it only functions effectively during deep sleep. A groundbreaking 2013 study in *Science* revealed that during sleep, channels in the brain expand, allowing cerebrospinal fluid to perform a "wash cycle," clearing out metabolic waste, including the amyloid-beta plaques associated with Alzheimer's disease [9]. During sleep, your brain also consolidates memories, regulates key hormones like cortisol and insulin, and repairs cellular damage. You must become a fierce protector of your sleep hygiene. Go to bed and wake up at roughly the same time every day, even on weekends. This stabilizes your internal clock. Your bedroom should be like a cave: cool, dark, and quiet. For the last hour before bed, declare a moratorium on screens. The blue light they emit suppresses melatonin, your body's "sleep hormone" [10]. Instead, read a physical book, listen to calming music, or take a warm bath.

Stress Management: The "normal" life we described in the last chapter is a life bathed in a sea of chronic, low-grade stress. Your "freeze, fight, or flight" response is constantly activated, marinating your body in the stress hormone cortisol. This state accelerates every negative aging process. Learning to manage it is an essential medical intervention.

Again, your pets are your guides. After a startling noise, Sirius might bark, but a moment later, he gives a full-body shake—literally shaking it off—and comes over for a reassuring pat. Your cat Leo spends hours in a state of quiet, non-judgmental presence. They both show us that managing stress is about creating moments of deliberate "off-switching" to activate the "rest and digest" system. Find a simple, daily practice that works for you. Take five deep, slow breaths, focusing on a longer exhale. This has been shown to directly stimulate the vagus nerve, instantly calming your physiology [11]. Even a 10-minute walk in a green space has been demonstrated to lower cortisol levels and reduce anxious thoughts.

Conclusion: The Strategic Choice

The *Path to the Pillbox* is the path of least resistance. It is the default setting of modern life. If you do nothing—if you let the stress of caregiving consume your schedule, if you rely on processed food for convenience, and if you ignore your own blood pressure—gravity will pull you down that road. You will arrive at the destination of frailty and polypharmacy not because you chose it, but because you didn't choose to stop it.

The *Path to Fewer Pills, More Paws* is different. It requires a choice. It demands engagement.

The High-5 strategy—strengthening your **Physical** body, fueling with **Nutritional** precision, maintaining **Vascular** flow, building **Cognitive & Social** reserve, and prioritizing **Restorative Health**—is not a list of chores. It is a declaration of independence from the pillbox.

It acknowledges that while we cannot stop time, we can change how we travel through it. It accepts that if your arteries are stiffening, the answer lies not just in a prescription, but in movement that pushes blood to the brain. It understands that if your mind feels overloaded, the remedy is not just "pushing through," but respecting the biological necessity of sleep and connection.

This path is about giving your fifty-five-year-old body what it truly needs, rather than just treating the symptoms of what it lacks.

And sometimes, the best way to do that is to look at the simple wisdom in your own living room. Look at Sirius. He doesn't obsess over the data. He simply lives the protocol. He moves with purpose (Physical). He rests deeply without guilt

(Restorative). He engages with you with total focus (Social). He is the master of Healthspan because he never worries about his lab results.

You now have the flipped map. You know the biology. By investing in your own health today, you are ensuring that you will be strong enough, clear enough, and resilient enough to be the Conductor your family needs for the journey ahead.

Now that we have secured your foundation, it is time to turn our attention back to the daily logistics of caring for Barbara. In the next section, we will open the "Conductor's Toolkit" and give you the specific scripts, checklists, and systems to manage the chaos of the healthcare system itself.

PART 4 | THE TOOLKIT

Mastering the Orchestra

This section is the tactical heart of your transformation into a proactive care partner. Having understood the biological changes in your full house, and the system you are up against, you are now ready to step into your role as the **Conductor**. These chapters provide the hands-on systems, scripts, and checklists you need to manage the most challenging aspects of your parent's care with clarity, confidence, and compassion.

Auditioning the Orchestra

You are standing in your mother's bathroom, looking for a Band-Aid, when the sight stops you in your tracks.

The medicine cabinet is a chaotic jumble of amber plastic. There is a bottle of lisinopril from six months ago sitting next to a new prescription for losartan. There are two different calcium supplements, expired eye drops, a tube of antifungal cream, and a small dish of loose pills whose identity is a complete mystery.

This isn't just clutter. It's a cacophony.

Right now, your parent's healthcare is an orchestra playing without a leader. The cardiologist is playing loud and fast to keep the heart pumping. The rheumatologist is blasting away for the arthritis. The primary care doctor is trying to play a steady melody for blood pressure. Separately, they are all talented musicians. But together? They are making a racket.

And the person suffering from the noise is your parent.

It is time for you to step up to the podium. You are the Conductor. You do not need a medical degree to do this; you simply need to recognize that the current volume is too loud, and it is time to bring order to the performance.

The Sound Check

Before we can fix the music, we have to know exactly who is playing. In the pharmacy world, we call this the "Brown Bag Review."

The next time you visit Barbara, bring a large, empty paper grocery bag. Your goal is to be exhaustive. You need to gather **everything**. Most medication errors happen in the gray zones between what the doctor *thinks* she is taking and what she is *actually* taking.

The Prescription Bottles: Check the nightstand, the bathroom, the purse, and the kitchen counter.

The OTC Section: Dig through the drawers. Grab the aspirin, the ibuprofen (Advil), the cold remedies, and the antacids.

The Supplements: Grab the giant bottle of Vitamin D, the fish oil, and the turmeric capsules her neighbor recommended.

The "Occasional" Players: Do not forget the eye drops, the creams, the inhalers, and the patches.

Now, dump them all onto the dining room table. This pile is the current score. Look at it honestly. Is it a harmonious melody? Or is it a chaotic mess of fifteen different instruments fighting for air?

Transcribing the Score

We need to turn that chaos into a document of pure clarity. Open **The Master Medication List** template (**Appendix 1**) or see the table in **Figure 8.1** below. You are going to create a table with five crucial columns. This will become your sheet music.

1. **Medication Name:** Write down exactly what is on the bottle. Crucially, include both the **Brand** and **Generic** names (e.g., *Lipitor / Atorvastatin*). This prevents the most common medical error: confusing two names for the same drug.

2. **Dose & Form:** Is it a 10 mg tablet? A 50 mcg patch? Precision is essential here. A small change in numbers can mean a massive change in effect.

3. **Instructions:** Copy the instructions exactly. "Take one tablet by mouth twice daily with meals." Include those other details—*with meals, at bedtime.*

4. **Prescriber:** Who ordered this? Was it Dr. Evans (Primary) or Dr. Jones (Urology)? You need to know who is directing this particular instrument so you know who to call when there is a problem.

5. **The "Why" (Indication):** This is the Conductor's most important rule: **If there is an instrument on stage, you must know why it is there.** Ask Barbara, *"Mom, what is this pill for?"* If neither of you knows—if the answer is *"Dr. Evans added it years ago"*—circle it in red. That is a musician sitting on stage who doesn't know the song. That is your first lead for the doctor.

Spotting the Discord

With your sheet music written out, you can now look for the places where the music clashes. You don't need to be a pharmacist to spot the four most common types of discord.

Figure 8.1. Medication Table
from the Master Medication List Template
(Full Version can be found in Appendix 1)

All templates & forms can also be found in the **Caregiver's Toolkit**
@ **www.myrxpro.com/caregivers-toolkit**

Patient Name:_______________________________________

Date Updated: _______________________________________

Allergies: _______________________________________

Part 1: The Master Medication List

Medication Name	Dose	Instructions	Prescriber	What its for?
Brand & Generic	e.g., 10 mg	How and When	Who Ordered it?	The Why
Example: Glucophage/ Metformin	1000 mg	Take 1 with Breakfast and Dinner	Dr. Frost	Diabetes

PART 2: The Pharmacist's Triage (Red Flag Check)

Review your completed list above. Look for these "Red Flags"

◯ **Duplication:** Is she taking two drugs for the same thing? (e.g., Aleve AND Ibuprofen?) .

◯ **The Cascade:** Is she taking a drug to fix the side effect of another drug? (e.g., Taking a bladder pill because a water pill makes her pee?) .

◯ **Beers List Risks:** Is she taking "PM" sleep aids (Benadryl/Diphenhydramine) or Benzodiazepines (Xanax/Ativan)?

🍄 Pharmacist Pro Tip! 🍄

STOP!

Before you crush that pill: If it has 'ER' or 'XR' on the label, crushing it turns a 24-hour dose into a 1-second overdose.

Always ask your pharmacist: 'Is this safe to crush?'

Many medications designed for older adults are "Extended Release" (look for ER, XR, SR, or CD next to the name). These pills contain a massive dose meant to dissolve slowly over 24 hours. If you crush them, you break that time-release mechanism, dumping the entire 24-hour dose into their system instantly. This can cause dangerous sedation, a sudden drop in blood pressure, or worse.

On the other hand, if the pill is "scored"—has a line etched down the middle—that generally means it can be split and crushed. If you do not know, DO NOT CRUSH A PILL without talking to your pharmacist first. If swallowing is an issue, ask the pharmacist if the medication comes in a liquid form, a patch, or a version that is safe to crush.

Duplication:

Sometimes, two doctors unwittingly order the same instrument, or a patient takes a generic version alongside the brand name. Is she taking *Lipitor* in the morning and *atorvastatin* at night? She is playing the same note twice, risking an overdose. Is she taking *Aleve* (naproxen) for her knees and *Advil* (ibuprofen) for her back? These two NSAID drummers are banging on the same kidney. It is simply too much noise.

The Prescribing Cascade

As discussed in detail in Chapter 6, the Prescribing Cascade is the most insidious pattern in geriatrics. It happens when a side effect of Drug A is misinterpreted as a *new disease*, leading to the prescription of Drug B.

Mom starts a blood pressure pill. Two weeks later, her ankles swell (a common side effect). Instead of adjusting the first pill, the doctor adds a diuretic to fix the swelling. The diuretic makes her pee all night, ruining her sleep. So, the doctor adds a bladder pill.

Scan your list. Is there a drug here that is treating the side effect of another drug?

The Beers Criteria

Some medications are simply too harsh for an older body. The American Geriatrics Society tracks these on the "Beers Criteria," a list of drugs that carry more risk than benefit for seniors. Last updated in 2023, a link to the full paper and any future updates, can be found at MyRxPro.com.

The Anticholinergics: The "PM" Sleep Aids or drowsy Antihistamines. The number one offender is **diphenhydramine** (Benadryl, Tylenol PM). In an 84-year-old, it blocks the brain chemicals needed for memory, causing confusion and delirium.

The Benzodiazepines: Drugs like **Xanax** and **Ativan** dampen the central nervous system. They slow the body's tempo down so much that the risk of falling increases by up to 50%.

> ### ♀ Pharmacist Pro Tip! ♀
>
> **A Critical Warning: The Medication-Dementia Link**
> This is one of the most urgent findings in geriatric science from the last decade. There is now significant evidence that long-term use of **Anticholinergic** and **Benzodiazepine** medications is associated with a higher risk of developing dementia.
> For years, we warned against these drugs in older adults because of side effects like falls and confusion. The new evidence suggests the risk is far graver and more permanent. This makes the deprescribing of these drugs not just a good idea for improving quality of life, but a critical mission for long-term brain protection.

"As Needed" Mystery

In medicine, we call these "PRN" medications. But without clear rules, improvisation is dangerous. If Barbara has an opioid for pain "as needed," what does that mean? Every four hours? Only when the pain is severe? Without strict parameters, she might accidentally stack sedatives on a difficult night. Circle every "As Needed" drug. Your note for the doctor is simple: *We need clear rules for this.*

You may look at Barbara's Medication List and think, *"I just wrote down a bunch of words, but I don't understand any of it. Is Amlodipine for her heart or her kidneys? Is Gabapentin making her sleepy?"* That is a perfectly natural thought, but let's explore where you should and shouldn't look for answers.

Paging Dr Google!

You have reviewed the orchestra. You have looked for the discord. Now, what do you do?

First, **do not stop any medication on your own.** Abruptly stopping a beta-blocker or a sedative can be medically dangerous. You are the Conductor, but you still need the composers—the doctors—to rewrite the score.

Your instinct will be to open your phone and ask Dr. Google. **Resist that urge.**

Here is why you cannot "Google" or use Artificial Intelligence to get your way out of polypharmacy:

If you search for "Side effects of Lisinopril," you will get a list of 50 terrifying possibilities, from a mild cough to instant death. Algorithms don't know your mother's kidney function, her weight, or her history. They lack the one thing you have: The Baseline. Only a human pharmacist can blend the data with the human context.

An online interaction checker will flag a "Major Interaction" between two drugs that Barbara has taken safely for ten years. It just knows what it was programmed with. Which, again, is the problem, it's programmed to avoid a lawsuit, not to be a care partner's ally.

AI-based interaction checkers also cannot account for your mother's kidney function, her weight loss, her over-the-counter medications, or the ten-year history her pharmacist carries in their head. For these reasons, AI can be your starting point for questions, but not your final authority for decisions.

You will end up terrified to give her the morning pills, but ultimately, the decision to stop requires the decision of a physician. What if you stopped but it's the withdrawal symptoms that are dangerous? Knowing what to ask Dr Google and AI is one thing, but how do you ask what you don't know?

Instead, consult your pharmacist. You need a human filter.

Consult the Pharmacist

The pharmacist is the most accessible healthcare provider in the system. You don't need a co-pay, and they are the only ones who see the *entire* picture across all specialists.

They are your decoder. They speak "Doctor," but they explain it in "English."

Want to level up that medication review? Don't just bring your list, bring the Brown Bag to the pharmacy. Schedule a "Brown Bag Review" with the pharmacist. This is a standard term in pharmacy; most pharmacists know what this is.

Just as before, put *every* bottle (prescription, vitamin, herbal, eye drop) into a bag. Go to the pharmacy at a slow time (usually mid-morning, Tuesday through Thursday). Avoid Monday mornings or late afternoons. Retail pharmacies are understaffed (efficiency). If you can help it, do not just show up. Call ahead and ask: 'What is the best time for a 15-minute consultation?' If they cannot do it, ask for a scheduled appointment. Say, *"I am auditing my mother's medication list for her doctor's appointment. Can you help me flag the priorities?"*

Do not ask, *"What does this pill do?"* (That gets you the generic speech). Ask these three strategic questions to arm yourself for the doctor:

1. **"Is this a Prescribing Cascade?"** Say, "I noticed she is taking a water pill (Furosemide) and also a pill for low

potassium. Is the water pill *causing* the low potassium?" The pharmacist can confirm if Pill B is only there to fix Pill A.

2. **"Is this dose renal-adjusted?"** Say, "My mom is 85 and frail. Is this the standard adult dose, or is it the geriatric dose?" Many seniors are on doses designed for 40-year-old men. The pharmacist can instantly spot if she is effectively overdosing because her kidneys act their age.

3. **"If we wanted to deprescribe, what is the safest order?"** Say, "If the doctor agrees to reduce her burden, which one should go first? And does it need a taper?" You never stop a drug alone. But knowing that *"The Benzo needs a 3-month taper, but the Statin can stop today"* gives you a roadmap to present to the doctor.

By consulting the pharmacist *before* the doctor's visit, you are no longer walking in with vague worries. You are walking in with clinical questions.

Instead of saying, *"I think she takes too many pills,"* you are saying, *"The pharmacist noted that her Gabapentin dose is high for her kidney function. Can we review that?"*

The doctor cannot ignore the second question. You have used the pharmacist to turn your Medication List into "Clinical Data."

Conclusion: The New Score

You gave that pharmacist a 'Leo' elbow nudge. You gave them the structural permission they needed to step out of their fast-paced workflow and use their extensive expertise to be your ally. You were the friction that slowed down the machinery. You forced the system to pay attention to Barbara.

When you walk into that next appointment with Barbara, you won't be fumbling through a bag of bottles or trying to remember if the blue pill is taken with breakfast or dinner. You will be holding a red-lined Master Score. You are offering the doctor the clarity they lack, and the questions they need to hear.

You have moved from being a helpless audience member to the leader of the band. You are no longer just the daughter; you are the Conductor. And when you control the noise, Barbara finally gets to live in harmony.

9 | The 8-Minute Appointment

A System for Leading with Clarity, Confidence, and Compassion

The cardiologist's appointment for your mother, Barbara, has been on your calendar for two months, a small square of impending stress. You've arranged to leave work early and confirmed transportation. But underneath the logistics, a real anxiety is churning. You have a nagging feeling that her new blood pressure medication is making her dizzy, but you don't know how to bring it up. Last time, you left feeling rushed, unheard, and clutching an "After Visit Summary" that felt like it had been assembled by a four-year-old with a pair of safety scissors—a chaotic mishmash of old diagnoses, new instructions, and lab orders for six months from now.

You felt lost in the system. Today, we change that.

This chapter provides your system for transforming the modern medical encounter from a source of frustration into an opportunity for productive partnership. As we've discussed, the healthcare landscape has changed. Your doctor is operating under immense time pressure. The key to being heard is not to talk louder, but to talk with impeccable clarity and preparation. This system will turn you from a passive spectator into the respected, prepared leader of your parent's care team. The mission is to be the friction—to slow down the fast machinery of the healthcare system and force it to pay attention to Barbara. While we have its attention, we must be efficient; this is why we prepare.

Preparation is Power

The outcome of an eight-minute appointment is decided in the thirty minutes you spend preparing at home. This is where you marshal your facts and define your mission. Your goal is to create one simple, powerful document: your **One-Page Briefing** (Appendix 2) and **Figure 9.1**.

The One-Page Briefing

This single piece of paper is your conductor's baton. It commands attention; when the conductor raises that baton everyone's eyes are on the conductor. It brings order to chaos and immediately signals to the doctor that you are a serious partner, not just a worried observer.

First, you must ruthlessly prioritize. You cannot solve every problem in one visit. If you try to address twelve issues, you will likely solve none of them. Instead, triage your concerns down to the **Top 3 Priorities**. This focuses the entire conversation before it even begins. The exception is safety; safety is always a priority. Your list shouldn't be vague; it should be actionable. For example:

1. *Discuss dizziness since starting amlodipine; explore alternatives.*
2. *Ask about safer options for managing arthritis pain.*
3. *Request a referral for a hearing test.*

Figure 9.1. The One-Page Briefing Template, part 1

(Full Version can be found in Appendix 2)

All templates & forms can also be found in the **Caregiver's Toolkit**
@ **www.myrxpro.com/caregivers-toolkit**

This One-Page Briefing template to be used before every doctor's appointment to ensure the 8-minute visit is efficient and productive. Hand this One-Page Briefing to the doctor immediately upon entering the room. *"I've put together a one-page summary with our main goals and an updated medication list on the back."*

Patient Name: ____
Appointment Date: ____
Physician: ____

Do not walk in with a laundry list. Triage your concerns down to the three most urgent issues. If it's not on this list, it waits for next time.

I. The "Top 3" Priorities
Priority #1: ____
Example: "Discuss dizziness since starting amlodipine."

Priority #2: ____
Example: "Explore safer options for arthritis pain."

Priority #3: ____
Example: "Request referral for hearing test."

Figure 9.2 The One-Page Briefing Template
parts 2 & 3

(Full Version can be found in Appendix 2)

All templates & forms can also be found in the **Caregiver's Toolkit**
@ www.myrxpro.com/caregivers-toolkit

II. The Data (Not Drama)

For each priority above, list specific, observable facts.
Avoid vague statements like "She seems dizzy."
Use dates, times, and specific incidents.

Observation Log for Priority #1:

When:____

What Happened:____

Frequency:____

Triggers: (e.g. after morning pills:)_____________________

Observation Log for Priority #2:

Details:____

III. The Attachments

Have these important document ready in case they are needed:

○ **Updated Master Medication List** (Includes ALL pills, vitamins, OTCs).
○ **Recent Blood Pressure/Blood Sugar Logs** (if applicable).
○ **Any other relevant charts, logs, or journals** (e.g., weight, symptoms)

Data, Not Drama

Doctors struggle with vague complaints. A statement like *"Mom seems dizzy sometimes"* is not useful clinical data—it's just noise. To be an effective partner, you must transform your subjective worry into objective facts. Under that first goal on your briefing sheet, write exactly what you saw:

"Dizziness Log: Noticed dizziness 3x this week (Mon PM, Tues AM, Thurs PM). Each time was when standing up from her chair about 1–2 hours after her morning pills. Had to hold onto the wall to steady herself on Tuesday."

Do you see the difference? You have just handed the doctor a pattern, not a feeling.

The Attachments

The non-negotiable foundation of this briefing is the **Master Medication List** you created. Print out a clean, updated copy and staple it to the back. Attach your logs, journals, records, and any other supporting documents. This helps to give a baseline for Barbara. A minute the doctor spends searching for the data is a minute they are not thinking about Barbara. If you don't know, ask the doctor, *"Is there any data you want us to bring back for the 6-month appointment?"*

Execution: A Masterclass in Medical Communication

You've done the prep work. Now it's time to execute the plan with calm confidence.

The Opening Gambit

The moment the doctor enters the room, the clock is ticking.

This first thirty seconds will set the tone. As you shake their hand, hand them your One-Page Briefing. Say, *"Dr. Evans, thank you for seeing us. To help make this visit as efficient as possible, we've put together a one-page summary with our main goals and an updated medication list on the back."*

You have changed the dynamic from reactive to collaborative. You've shown profound respect for their time and given them a clear roadmap. You now have their full attention. The electronic medical record is designed to guide the doctor through a billing checklist. Your One-Page Briefing disrupts that algorithm. It forces the human being in the white coat to look at the human being in the chair.

The Annual Wellness Visit

If your goal is a big-picture, holistic review, a standard follow-up may not be the right venue. Your secret weapon is the **Medicare Annual Wellness Visit (AWV)**. This yearly appointment is specifically designed for a longer, comprehensive conversation focused on prevention and medication reconciliation.

When you call to schedule the AWV, say, *"I'd like to schedule my mother, Barbara's, Annual Wellness Visit. We want to do a full review of her medications and health goals."*

This appointment is a protected, longer time slot tailor-made for the proactive, goal-setting conversation this book champions.

Navigating Hard Conversations

Raising a concern can feel confrontational, but the key is to frame it as a collaborative inquiry rather than a complaint.

Let's look at how to handle that dizziness from the new blood pressure medication. First, **lead with the data** you collected. You might say: "Dr. Evans, as you can see from our sheet, I've been tracking her dizzy spells specifically since she started the new amlodipine."

Next, **state the shared goal** to diffuse any defensiveness. You want to remind them you are on the same team: "My absolute top priority is preventing a fall. I know that's your goal, too. I'm just concerned the dizziness is putting her at high risk."

Finally, **inquire collaboratively.** Show you've done your homework, but ask for their expertise to solve the puzzle: "Given that the latest guidelines suggest a blood pressure goal under 130 is appropriate, and Mom is running around 115 on this dose, would you be open to exploring our options? Perhaps a lower dose might give us a 'sweet spot' where her blood pressure is managed, but her fall risk is lower."

Ensuring Clarity with the "Teach-Back" Method

Finally, do not leave the room until you have closed the loop.

We have all experienced the "Parking Lot Panic"—that moment you buckle your seatbelt, turn to your parent, and ask, *"So, did he say to start the new pill today or tomorrow?"* only to be met with a blank stare.

To prevent this, borrow a technique from the very best medical professionals: **The "Teach-Back" Method.**

In pharmacy school, we teach to ask patients to repeat instructions back to us to ensure they understand. As the Conductor, you are going to flip the script. You are going to "teach back" the plan to the doctor to ensure *you* understand.

See **Figure 9.3** below for a template to help get you started. This template can also be found in **Appendix 3**.

It doesn't need to be formal. In fact, a little humility works wonders here. As the doctor reaches for the doorknob, simply say:

"Doctor, thank you. Just so I am 100% certain I've got this right—and so I don't mess it up when we get home—let me repeat the plan back to you..."

Then, look at your notes and list the changes:

1. *"We are cutting the amlodipine to 2.5 mg starting tomorrow."*
2. *"We are stopping the Lisinopril completely."*
3. *"And we are booking a blood pressure check in two weeks."*
4. *"Did I miss anything?"*

This 30-second conversation is the most valuable part of the entire visit. If you heard "20 mg" but the doctor meant "10 mg," this is the only chance to catch that error before it becomes a medical emergency. When the doctor says, *"Yes, you've got it,"* you aren't just leaving with a prescription; you are leaving with certainty. If they are rushing, say *"I need 30 seconds to read this back for safety"*—the word 'safety' usually stops a doctor in their tracks.

The Follow-Through: Where the Plan Becomes Reality

The appointment doesn't end when you walk out the door. In fact, the most critical moment for safety often happens five minutes later, in the quiet of your car. This is where you cement the gains you just made.

Figure 9.3 The Teach Back Template

(Full Version can be found in Appendix 3)

All templates & forms can also be found in the **Caregiver's Toolkit** @ **www.myrxpro.com/caregivers-toolkit**

Use this template script at the end of the appointment to ensure you understand the new plan.

"Let me repeat the plan back to you..."

Medication Changes: *Cut amlodipine to 2.5mg starting tomorrow. Stop Lisinopril*

New To-Dos: *Monitor BP twice a week. Call office in 2 weeks.*

Next Appointment: *Make another appointment in 6 weeks*

Other concerns discussed: *Call about the lab work next week*

Is there anything that I missed?

First, Tame the Paperwork Monster. On your way out, you were likely handed an "After Visit Summary" (AVS). It may also be found in the Patient Portal. Let's be honest about what this document really is: it is a liability shield designed by lawyers, not a guidebook designed for care partners. In modern healthcare, the AVS has become a bloated, ten-page jumble of automated safety warnings and billing codes. The critical information you actually need is in there, but it is often sprinkled like breadcrumbs through pages of legal fluff.

Do not let it overwhelm you. Your job is to ignore 90% of the boilerplate and find the vital 10%.

Compare the AVS against the notes you took during the "Teach-Back." Find the section usually labeled "Orders" or "Medication Changes." Does it match what you heard? If it does, grab your notebook and scribble a clean, three-point **"After-Action Report"** that cuts through the noise. It should look something like this:

- **Med Change:** *Amlodipine now 2.5mg daily (start tomorrow). Stop Lisinopril.*
- **To Do:** *Pick up new Rx. Call pharmacy to confirm old Rx is canceled.*
- **Monitor:** *Check for dizziness daily. Check BP twice a week.*
- **Follow-up:** *Send update via portal on Nov 15th.*

Next, Close the Loop with the Pharmacist. This is the step most people skip, and it is where errors happen. Do not assume the doctor's computer successfully talked to the pharmacy's computer. Be the bridge.

Call your regular pharmacist—your safety net—and loop them in verbally:

"Hi, this is Barbara's son. We just saw Dr. Evans. He has discontinued her lisinopril and is sending over a new prescription for amlodipine. We're actually starting at a half-dose of 2.5mg. I just wanted to give you a heads-up so you can double-check everything when it comes through."

> ♟ **Pharmacist Pro Tip!** ♟
>
> ### The "One Pharmacy Rule"
>
> You might fill a heart med at the big-box store because it's cheaper, grab an antibiotic at the local grocery store because it's faster, and get specialized dementia meds via mail order.
>
> **This is dangerous**. Pharmacists have computer systems designed to catch lethal drug interactions—but they only work if they know everything your parent is taking. If you split prescriptions between three pharmacies, none of those safety nets are working.
>
> The insurance company may try to steer you to different pharmacies to save themselves pennies. You must resist this fragmentation. Safety requires a single pair of eyes on the entire list.
>
> Pick one pharmacy and stick to it for everything. The safety of having one professional overseeing the entire regimen outweighs saving a few dollars on co-pays.

Finally, Update the Master List. When you get home, update your Master Medication List immediately. An out-of-date medication list is a dangerous document. If the paramedics arrive next week and you hand them the old list, they will treat her based on yesterday's reality. I suggest at least 3 copies, one for the hospital "go-bag" we will discuss in later chapters, one for the fridge (if privacy allows) with the POLST form, and the last one for you to bring to appointments or to show the pharmacist.

The Power of the Portal. A few weeks later, use the patient portal to close the loop with the doctor. You don't need another appointment; you just need to confirm the plan is working. Keep it brief and data-driven:

"Dear Dr. Evans, per our visit on Oct 28, here is an update on Barbara. Since reducing her amlodipine, her dizzy spells have resolved completely. Home BP readings are stable around 135/80. Please confirm if we should continue this 2.5mg dose. Thank you."

Conclusion: Interrupting the 8-minute appointment

By building the Medication List, auditing the "Why" behind every pill, and consulting the pharmacist, you have done something the system rarely does: you have looked at Barbara as a whole person, not a collection of failing organs.

You are no longer walking into the doctor's office with a vague sense that "something is wrong." You are walking in with data. You are walking in with a red-lined score. You are walking in with the quiet confidence of someone who knows the truth about what happens at your kitchen table when the clinic is closed.

It is scary to challenge the status quo, but the default path leads to polypharmacy, adverse drug events, and the prescribing cascade.

A Data-Driven Framework for the Hardest Conversations

When Barbara drives, do you find yourself pressing your right foot hard against the floor as if it's a phantom brake pedal? Do you grip the door handle until your knuckles turn white?

Picture this: Barbara pulls out into traffic, causing another driver to slam on their brakes and blare their horn. She doesn't seem to notice. On the way to the grocery store, she drives ten miles under the speed limit, drifting slightly into the other lane. When parking, she misjudges the distance and gently bumps the concrete stop, jarring both of you.

She laughs it off—*"Whoops, this car is bigger than I remember."* But you are not laughing. You feel a cold, sickening knot of dread in your stomach. You know, with a certainty that terrifies you, that her driving is no longer safe.

The Dual Threats to Independence

Two of the greatest safety issues that threaten Barbara's long-term independence are falls and no longer being able to safely drive. Both of these realities come with massive emotional barriers that make them incredibly difficult to address.

Of all the difficult roles a care partner is asked to play, this is perhaps the hardest. Confronting a parent about driving—or their ability to safely walk around their own home—can feel like a betrayal. These activities are not just about transportation or mobility; they are about freedom, competence, and adulthood. To challenge them is to challenge the very core of who they are.

Most of these confrontations go poorly because we start them from a place of raw emotion: *"Mom, you have to stop driving!"* This approach, born of love and fear, is almost guaranteed to be met with anger, denial, and a breakdown in trust. It becomes a battle of wills, a fight you are unlikely to win.

There is a different way. We can transform this emotional power struggle into a calm, objective process. It is about removing your personal opinion from the equation and instead building an irrefutable case based on facts. You will move from being the "bad guy" to being the lead investigator for "Operation: Safe At Home".

The Rule: Data First, Discussion Second

The reason these conversations feel impossible is that we almost always start them from the wrong place—our feelings.

"Mom, I'm terrified to be in the car with you." "Dad, I don't think you should be living alone anymore."

These statements, while true, are immediately interpreted as personal attacks on their competence. The response is predictably defensive: *"I'm a perfectly good driver!"* You are now in an argument, and you have already lost.

The solution is to fundamentally change your approach. Your new mantra is: **Data first, discussion second**. Before you have "The Big Talk," you must go on a mission to gather clear, objective, undeniable evidence.

Let's use driving as the quintessential example of how to build this case.

Phase 1: Intelligence Gathering

For the next few weeks, your job is to become a silent, non-judgmental observer. This is not about criticizing; it is about collecting facts. Research consistently shows that discussions about driving are most successful when based on specific, observable behaviors rather than general assumptions [1].

Find excuses to ride in the passenger seat. While you are there, log specific events with dates and times using the **Safety & Driving Observation Log** (See Appendix 5 and Figure 10.1 below). Look for the key warning signs identified by geriatrics experts [2, 3]:

- **Close Calls:** Did another driver have to brake or swerve?
- **Vehicle Control:** Was there drifting, abrupt braking, or dangerously slow speeds?
- **Cognitive Gaps:** Did she get lost on a familiar route or miss a traffic signal?
- **Physical Evidence:** Are there new, unexplained dings or scrapes on the car?

Think of this as the "Leo Framework." Your cat, Leo, doesn't complain that his legs feel weak. He just shows you. He crouches to jump, hesitates, and then chooses the ottoman instead. That hesitation is pure data. Your parent won't announce, "My reaction time has slowed," but their driving will show you. Your job is to capture that data without judgment.

Figure 10.1. The Safety & Driving Observation Log, part 1
(Full Version can be found in Appendix 5)

All templates & forms can also be found in the **Caregiver's Toolkit** @ **www.myrxpro.com/caregivers-toolkit**

Use this log to track specific, objective events over a 2-week period. Be a "silent observer" like your cat, Leo. Do not critique in the moment; simply record the data. This document is your evidence for the doctor.

Part 1: The Driving Log
*Ride as a passenger. Watch for: **Close Calls** (braking/swerving), **Vehicle Control** (drifting/abrupt braking/slow speed) **Cognitive Gaps** (getting lost/missed a traffic sign/delayed reaction)*

Date & Time	Event Type (Check One)	Description of Incident (Be Specific)
Ex: 10/14, 2pm	◯ Close Call ◯ Confusion ◯ Control	*Drifted into left lane on Main St; oncoming car honked.*

Phase 2: Building Your Coalition

You should not do this alone. Trying to be the sole enforcer can permanently damage your relationship. Instead, involve your siblings or trusted relatives to create a consensus. This prevents "triangulation," where a parent might pit one child against another [4].

Most importantly, empower the doctor. A direct recommendation from a physician is the single most influential factor in an older adult's decision to stop driving.

But the doctor cannot act without evidence. Schedule an appointment and use your **One-Page Briefing** (Appendix 2) to present your logs. The doctor will need this information to make a decision.

"Dr. Evans, our goal today is to discuss Mom's driving. My siblings and I have been keeping a log of specific incidents, which I've summarized here. We would be grateful for your professional assessment and help in having this difficult conversation."

You have now made the doctor your most powerful ally, equipping them with the clinical data needed to write a prescription for safety.

Phase 3: The Conversation and The Tactical Pause

When the time comes to talk, the goal is not to "win," but to solve a problem. Frame it with love:

"Mom, we need to have a hard conversation, and I want you to know it's coming from a place of deep love. My number one goal is to have you with us, safe and healthy, for many more years."

Then, present the data calmly:

"Last Tuesday, on the way to the store, we had that close call where the other car had to swerve. And when we looked at the car yesterday, we saw this new scrape on the bumper. These are the kinds of things that worry me."

Finally, pivot immediately to the solution. The conversation isn't about taking away the car; it's about replacing it with a **Mobility Plan** [5, 6].

"So, we've put together a plan. We set up a monthly fund for Uber or taxis. Mary will drive you on Wednesdays, and I'll take

you to bridge on Fridays. The goal is to make sure you can still go everywhere you love to go, just more safely."

You can do everything right, and your parent might still react with anger or denial: *"You're calling me incompetent! This is my life!"*

When this happens, do not argue back. Your mission now is to de-escalate. Use a **Tactical Pause**. The framework is simple: **Validate the Emotion + Re-state Your Intention + Initiate the Pause**.

"You're right to be angry. It sounds like you feel attacked, and that was not my intention. My only goal is to make sure you are safe because I love you. Why don't we pause this for now and just have a cup of tea?"

If they express hurt:

"I hear how hurt you are, and I am so sorry. It must feel awful to think I don't trust you. Please know this isn't about trust; it's about the fact that I couldn't live with myself if something happened to you. Let's not talk about it anymore today."

The tactical pause is not giving up. It is a strategic retreat that allows the emotional storm to pass, giving you the space to try again later—perhaps with your doctor ally in the room.

Extending the Framework

This same **Data → Allies → Conversation** framework applies to almost any safety crisis.

If you find burnt pans, keep a log (Data). Then suggest a meal delivery service not as a criticism, but as a convenience (Conversation). If you see them struggling to walk, note the frequency (Data). Then ask the doctor to order a home safety evaluation from an Occupational Therapist (Ally). Frame it as a "Safety Tune-Up" to keep them independent (Conversation).

Falls and Fear of the "Furniture Walkers"

While we are talking about the car keys, we need to talk about the carpet. Falls are the number one cause of injury and death in older adults, but they rarely happen out of the blue. Long before the ambulance is called, there are subtle, silent signals that stability is failing. The most common signal is **"Furniture Walking."**

Watch Barbara navigate her living room. Does she walk freely across the open space? Or does she subtly cruise from the back of the sofa, to the armchair, to the sideboard, trailing her hand on each item for balance? If she is connecting the dots of furniture to get across the room, she has lost her "Balance Confidence."

She is terrified of falling, and that fear is actually *increasing* her risk. This is a well-documented medical spiral known as

Figure 10.2 Home Safety Log, part 2
(Full Version can be found in Appendix 5)

All templates & forms can also be found in the **Caregiver's Toolkit** @ **www.myrxpro.com/caregivers-toolkit**

Use this log to track specific, objective events over a 2-week period. Be a "silent observer" like your cat, Leo. Do not critique in the moment; simply record the data. This document is your evidence for the doctor.

Part 2: Home Safety Log
The same cognitive gaps that affect driving often show up at home first. Look for: **Burnt pans, unlocked doors, "furniture walking" (using furniture for balance), medical attention for injuries, falls, or unexplained bruises**

Date & Time	Observation	Why it concerns you
Ex: 11/2, 10pm	*Stove burner left on High.*	*Fire risk; Did not know who turned it on.*

Figure 10.3 The Home Safety Audit
part 1
(Full Version can be found in Appendix 8)

All templates & forms can also be found in the **Caregiver's Toolkit**
@ **www.myrxpro.com/caregivers-toolkit**

Creating a Safe Environment for the Full House

Instructions: Walk through your home with "Fresh Eyes." We are looking for areas where physics works against the safety of an older adult. Research as shown these are the dangers to look out for.

☑ **The Floors (The Terrain)**

◯ **Remove ALL Throw Rugs:**

These are the #1 trip hazard for walkers and shuffling gaits.
A catch of the toe can lead to a hip fracture.

> *Bonus:* Removing them also helps old dogs who slip on shifting fabrics.

◯ **Secure Cords:** Tape down lamp cords running across walkways.

Prevents entanglement and tripping.

Figure 10.4 The Home Safety Audit
part 2
(Full Version can be found in Appendix 8)

All templates & forms can also be found in the **Caregiver's Toolkit**
@ **www.myrxpro.com/caregivers-toolkit**

☑ **The Lighting (The Horizon)**

◯ **Motion-Sensor Nightlights:** Install in the hallway, bathroom, and bedroom.

- Prevents falls during late-night bathroom trips by providing visual cues for balance.

- *Bonus:* Helps pets with failing vision navigate without bumping into walls.

◯ **Reduce Glare:** Close blinds at sunset.

- Prevents "Sundowning" shadows that trigger confusion and visual hallucinations.

☑ **The Stairs (The High Risk Zone)**

◯ **Contrast Tape:** Place a strip of bright/neon tape on the edge of every step.

- Older eyes lose depth perception. The tape clearly defines where the step ends so she doesn't miss a riser.

- *Bonus:* Helps pets see the drop-off.

◯ **Double Handrails:** Ensure there are rails on *both* sides of the stairwell so they can use both arms for leverage.

The Cycle of Fear:

1. She feels unsteady, so she moves less to avoid a fall.
2. Moving less causes her muscles to weaken (sarcopenia) and her reaction time to slow.
3. Weaker muscles make her *more* likely to fall.
4. Eventually, she trips. Even if not injured, she becomes terrified and stops moving entirely.

Your job as the Conductor is to break this cycle before the fall happens, before the cycle can start. And the way to do it is to stop talking about "Safety" and start talking about "Training."

Getting the Athlete to Training

Nobody wants to hear *"Mom, you're frail, don't fall."* It sounds condescending. Instead, treat her like an elite athlete who needs a tune-up.

"Mom, I noticed you've been holding onto the furniture a bit more lately. That tells me your 'stabilizer muscles' are getting a little tired. I don't want you to limit your life. I want to get you a Personal Trainer (Physical Therapist) to target those specific muscles so you can walk confidently again. Let's ask Dr. Evans for a referral for 'Gait and Balance Training' so you can stay independent."

This removes the shame of "aging." It frames the intervention (Physical Therapy) as empowerment, not medicalization. It focuses on the goal she wants: **Independence**.

The Physics of Safety: Traction, Terrain, and Chemistry

When we look at fall prevention, we need to stop thinking about "being careful" and start thinking about physics. Gravity is relentless. It does not care how much you love your mother;

it only cares about friction and balance. To keep Barbara safe, we have to audit the three physical systems that keep her upright.

- **Traction:** An athlete would never step onto the field in loose, backless shoes. Yet we often let our parents walk around on hardwood floors in loose, backless slippers that are essentially fall-generating devices. Swap the backless slippers for "indoor shoes" or slippers with a closed heel and a rubber grip sole. She needs stability, not just warmth. Additionally, when was her last podiatry appointment? Painful, overgrown, or fungal toenails change the biomechanics of how she steps, forcing her to shift her weight in dangerous ways. Regular foot care is not a spa luxury; it is a stability requirement.

- **Terrain:** Your home environment is an obstacle course. You have adapted to it; she cannot. Throw rugs are the number one enemy of the shuffling foot. If a rug is not nailed down, it is a trip hazard. Remove them. Furthermore, proprioception (knowing where your body is in space) declines with age. If the hallway is dark, Barbara literally cannot tell where the floor ends. Install motion-sensor nightlights. She cannot balance if she cannot see the horizon. This has the added benefit of helping Sirius, whose night vision is also failing, but we do this primarily so Barbara can navigate her home with dignity. (See Figure 10.3 and Appendix 8 for a Home Safety Audit).

- **Chemistry:** Sometimes the environment is safe, but the internal gyroscope is spinning. If she is suddenly wobbly, do not assume it is just "aging." Audit the Master Medication List. Is she on a blood pressure pill that causes orthostatic hypotension (dizziness upon standing)? Is she taking a "PM" sleep aid that leaves her chemically hungover? Removing one "wobbly" pill is often more effective than installing a dozen grab bars.

Falls: Function Over Fear

Addressing falls doesn't have to be a dramatic confrontation. It is a series of small, practical adjustments—better shoes, brighter lights, a medication review, and "training" (PT). By catching the "Furniture Walking" early, you aren't just preventing a broken hip; you are preserving her confidence to move. And movement, as we know, is life.

Conclusion: The Loving Act of Data

These conversations are some of the most difficult. They are hard because they sit at the painful intersection of safety and autonomy. The natural tendency is to either avoid them until a crisis forces our hand, or to charge in with emotion and create a conflict that fractures our relationships.

This data-driven framework is your path through this difficult terrain. By meticulously gathering your facts, building a supportive coalition, and approaching the final conversation with solutions, you are doing more than just solving a safety problem.

You are honoring your parent's dignity by treating them as a rational partner in their own care. You are demonstrating that your actions are rooted not in a desire for control, but in a profound and abiding love that seeks only to keep them safe and well.

11 | THE UNFILTERED BRAIN

Not just Memory Loss

If you are reading this chapter, you have likely already survived the "Memory Phase" of this journey. You have navigated the repeated questions, the misplaced keys, and the confusion over names. That phase was difficult, but it was largely manageable with sticky notes and patience.

But now, the weather has changed. You have entered the "Behavior Phase."

Perhaps your polite mother has started swearing, or your gentle father threw a coffee mug because he couldn't find the bathroom. Maybe your mother is anxiously packing a bag for a trip that doesn't exist, or the evening pacing has turned into sudden shouting. You are standing in the wreckage of a difficult afternoon thinking: *This isn't memory loss. This is madness. And I don't know how to fix it.*

Let me reassure you: It is not madness. And you are not failing. It is simply biology.

To survive these behaviors—without feeling constantly defeated or sedating your loved one into oblivion—we have to stop looking at them through the lens of human logic and start looking at them through the lens of neurobiology. When you understand the science of the changing brain, you gain the ultimate tool. You stop reacting to the chaos and start conducting the environment.

The Gatekeeper and The Unfiltered Brain

To understand why your parent is acting out, you have to understand what the healthy human brain actually does for a living. We think its primary job is to *think*, but its most important job is actually to *ignore*.

A healthy adult brain acts as a sophisticated Gatekeeper, ruthlessly filtering out ninety-nine percent of incoming sensory data so you can focus on the one percent that matters [1]. Right now, your Gatekeeper is actively filtering out the hum of your refrigerator, the feeling of your shirt collar against your neck, and the shadows moving on the wall.

Dementia dismantles the Gatekeeper.

Imagine for a moment that your own filters vanished right now. Suddenly, the hum of the fridge sounds like a roaring jet engine. The patterned rug looks like snakes writhing on the floor. The tag on your shirt feels like a razor blade against your skin. The world is coming at you at maximum volume, unedited, unmuted, and terrifyingly immediate.

Your parent is experiencing sudden-onset, severe sensory processing failure. If someone walked up to you in that terrifying, noisy chaos and tried to force a spoon into your mouth, or suddenly grabbed your arm to pull off your shirt for a bath, what would you do? You would scream, or you might slap their hand away. You wouldn't do it because you were being "mean" or because you had forgotten who they were. You would do it because your **Amygdala**—the brain's ancient threat-detection center—is screaming that you are under attack, and you are defending yourself.

When your parent acts out, they are not giving you a hard time. They are *having* a hard time.

The Biological Map

One of the most isolating feelings for a care partner is reading a generic pamphlet about dementia and thinking, *"Wait, my dad isn't doing this. Is his disease wrong? Am I doing something wrong?"*

It is vital to know that "dementia" is just an umbrella term. Beneath that umbrella are several different diseases, and each one follows a distinctly different structural map.

If your parent has classic **Alzheimer's Disease** (the most common form), their brain is following a map called **Retrogenesis**. Coined by Dr. Barry Reisberg, this theory explains that the Alzheimer's brain shifts in the exact reverse order of how it originally developed [2]. It is a "Last In, First Out" system. The executive logic centers (the Prefrontal Cortex) that took twenty years to build are the first to lose their connections. But the ancient survival centers (the Amygdala and Brainstem) remain robust and active until the very end. Your logic no longer works because their logic center is offline, but their emotional radar is wide awake.

However, if your parent has a different diagnosis, they are following a different map:

- **Frontotemporal Dementia (FTD):** This disease impacts the social and inhibition centers at the very front of the brain early on, but spares the memory centers for a long time. You might have a parent with perfect memory who suddenly begins shoplifting, swearing, or losing empathy. It isn't a psychological breakdown; the structural "brakes" on their behavior have simply disconnected.

- **Lewy Body Dementia (LBD):** This disease disrupts the brain's transport lines with abnormal proteins, creating severe electrical and chemical instability. This causes profound, rapid fluctuations where a person can shift from perfectly lucid to unresponsive in a matter of hours, often accompanied by vivid hallucinations and Parkinson's-like stiffness [3].

- **Vascular Dementia (VaD):** Caused by mini-strokes or poor blood flow, this damages the deep "highways" connecting different parts of the brain. These individuals often have brilliant "islands of ability" surrounded by sudden deficits, and their brain change is usually a step-wise change rather than a smooth, gradual fade.

You are not doing it wrong. Their biology is simply following a different blueprint.

The GEMS® and Neurochemical States: Your Conductor's Baton

If the structural map dictates *which* parts of the brain are disconnected, the brain's chemistry dictates *how* the person functions in any given moment.

To help families navigate this fluctuating chemistry, Teepa Snow, a brilliant occupational therapist and leading dementia educator, revolutionized the conversation by developing the **GEMS® State Model** [4]. This model shifts the focus entirely from what is lost to what abilities remain. She chose gemstones because they are precious, unique, and simply require the right setting to shine.

By bridging Teepa's behavioral model with neurobiology—and borrowing a few familiar lessons from our pets—we can give you the exact tools you need to interact with these different states, regardless of which underlying disease your parent has. As the Conductor, you already know how to do this for your pets; now we just apply it to your parent.

- **The Diamond State (Cholinergic Fraying):** Diamonds are clear and sharp, but they are rigid. They heavily control their habits and environment to mask the fact that they are slipping. Biologically, this corresponds to the fluctuation of *Acetylcholine*, the chemical responsible for encoding new learning.
    - Think of Leo the cat. He is sharp and loves you, but it must be on his terms. If you abruptly move his litter box, he will protest loudly. When your parent is in a Diamond state, they need their routine protected and their competence validated, not a logical debate.
- **The Emerald State (Dopamine Fluctuations):** Emeralds are "On the Go" and communicative, but they miss safety cues. Here, *Dopamine*—which drives motivation—is fluctuating. If the signal loops, they might pack and unpack a purse endlessly because the brain's "Go" signal is firing without the "Stop" signal.
    - Think of Sirius the dog seeing a squirrel. He doesn't calculate the safety of running into the street; his brain just says *Go!* Your parent in this state lacks the executive brakes to check

themselves. You cannot argue with the "Go" signal; you must walk with them and gently redirect it.

- **The Amber State (Brake Failure):** Ambers are caught entirely in a moment of sensation. They are touching, tasting, and exploring everything with limited safety awareness. The brain is experiencing a drop in *GABA* (the brain's calming "Brake Fluid") while excitatory chemicals spike. They are chemically incapable of stopping an impulse.
  - Sirius is also our resident Amber. If he finds a discarded sandwich on the sidewalk, you don't argue with him about why it is dirty. You stop talking, lower your voice, and warmly trade him for a better, safer treat. Sensation and redirection win over logic every time.
- **The Ruby & Pearl States (The Primal Connections):** As the journey progresses, fine motor coordination changes, but gross motor strength remains. The Pearl state is hidden within, primarily functioning on the Brainstem's primal receptors for *Oxytocin* (comfort) and *Endorphins* (pain relief).
  - When Leo is curled up in a deep sleep, he connects with you through warmth, vibration, and purring. A Pearl connects through this exact same primal chemistry of safety, rhythm, and touch.

Empowering the Care Partner

Learning the science behind these shifting states isn't meant to overwhelm you; it is meant to bring you a profound sense of relief.

For months, you may have felt like you were failing because you couldn't reason with your parent. But you cannot reason with fluctuating Dopamine, and you cannot debate a vanishing supply of GABA.

Understanding your parent's neurochemistry allows you to extend grace to them, and just as importantly, to yourself. It gives you permission to let go of the guilt and stop trying to force their brain to work the way it used to.

Your job is not to fix the underlying structural map. Your job is simply to assess the state they are in *right now* and meet them there. When you finally accept the biology, the anger and the arguments naturally dissolve. You step off the battlefield because you realize there was never an enemy to fight—just a changing brain doing the best it can.

You have the tools. You know the biology. You are ready to step onto the podium as a compassionate Conductor. In the next chapter, we will look at exactly how to put this plan into physical practice using the Paws Protocol.

Caring for the Unfiltered Brain

In the last chapter, we established that your parent's neurochemistry and structural wiring are shifting. We cannot fix the underlying biology, and there is no pill that can magically rewire those disconnected pathways. However, we hold immense power to change the *Environment*.

If the logic centers of the brain (the Prefrontal Cortex) are offline, we must stop trying to use them. Instead, we must use the input ports that are still wide open: the Amygdala (which processes emotion) and the Somatosensory Cortex (which processes physical touch) remain highly active long after words fail.

To understand how to do this, we simply need to look at Leo the cat and Sirius the dog. Our pets do not have complex social filters, and they do not use human logic to manage their day. They live entirely in a world of raw sensory input and immediate emotional reactions. Yet, they navigate the world peacefully most of the time because we instinctively know how to approach them. We don't use long, logical sentences to calm a frightened Sirius; we use our tone, our touch, and our presence.

To communicate with your parent's Unfiltered Brain, we are going to apply this exact same wisdom through the **Paws Protocol**. This is how we bypass the broken logic centers and speak directly to the emotional chemistry that remains.

The Biology of Co-Regulation

We tend to think of our emotions as private, internal experiences, but biologically, emotions are highly contagious. This phenomenon is powered by a specialized network in your brain called *Mirror Neurons*. These remarkable neurons fire not only when you perform an action, but also when you simply *watch* someone else perform that same action [1].

In a healthy brain, the frontal cortex acts as a protective filter to help distinguish between "Me" and "You." It can observe a stressful situation and say, *"That person is stressed, but I am separate, and I am safe."* In the Unfiltered Brain of dementia, that protective boundary dissolves. Because the logical filter is gone, their Amygdala is left wide open, absorbing the emotional climate of the room instantly. If you walk into the room with high cortisol levels (stress), tight shoulders, and a furrowed brow, your parent's mirror neurons instantly download your stressful state. They don't logically think, *"My daughter seems stressed today."* Instead, their brain immediately feels, *"WE are in danger."* This is exactly why telling someone to "calm down" never works when you say it through gritted teeth. Your words might say "calm," but your mirror neurons are broadcasting "threat." And the brain's ancient threat-detection center always listens to the neurons over the words.

The Thermostat vs. The Thermometer

As the disease progresses, your parent loses the ability to self-soothe; their internal emotional cooling system is broken. They are often running hot, living in a state of near-constant, low-level panic.

To survive and thrive in this phase, you must stop being a *Thermometer* and become the *Thermostat*.

A thermometer has no control over its environment; it simply reflects the temperature around it. If your parent is hot and angry, a thermometer caregiver gets hot and angry right back. If they are frantic, you get frantic. The heat in the room just continues to escalate until an emotional explosion happens.

To successfully care for the Unfiltered Brain, you must be the Thermostat. You do not reflect the temperature; you *set* the temperature. You decide that the energy in the room needs to be calm, low, and slow, and you use your own well-regulated nervous system to actively bring the temperature down.

To do this, we manually turn down the dials on the thermostat using the **3 Ts: Tone, Touch, and Tempo**.

1. Tone: The Music of Safety: The Unfiltered Brain may lose the ability to process semantics (the actual dictionary meaning of words), but it becomes an absolute expert at processing *Prosody* (the music, pitch, and rhythm of speech). Biologically, the human brain is wired to interpret sound frequencies as survival signals. High-pitched, loud, or fast sounds (like a scream or a siren) instantly trigger the *Startle Reflex* in the brainstem. This releases cortisol and preps the body to fight. Conversely, low, resonant, rhythmic sounds (like a cello or a mother's hum) bypass the threat detection system and actively down-regulate the Amygdala [2].

When you speak to a healthy adult, they process *what* you say. When you speak to a parent with a changing brain, they process *how* you say it.

Leo offers us a beautiful lesson here with his purr. We know he purrs when he is happy, but cats also purr when they are injured or terrified. The specific, low-frequency vibration of a cat's purr (between 25 and 150 Hertz) has actually been shown to lower blood pressure and promote physical healing [3]. Leo literally uses the physics of sound to self-soothe.

When you consciously lower your voice to a deep, rhythmic hum for Barbara, you are doing the exact same thing. You are using sound vibration to physically calm her nervous system. Drop your pitch and speak from your chest, not your throat. This lower, resonant voice mimics the acoustic signature of safety. Even if she doesn't fully understand the word "Shower," your low, rhythmic tone tells her chemical system, *"You are safe with me."*

2. Touch: Connection over Control: If you look at a neurological map of how the brain processes physical sensation (a map called the Cortical Homunculus), the hands are massive. They have an incredibly strong, dense, and direct connection to the brain. This makes touch the fastest way to activate calming systems, but it also makes it high-stakes.

Light, feathery touches (like quickly brushing a crumb off their shoulder) stimulate nerve fibers that send "alert" signals. To a sensory-sensitive brain, this feels like a bug landing on them, triggering an immediate pull-away reflex. However, firm, steady pressure stimulates deep receptors that release

Oxytocin—the brain's powerful chemical of connection and trust.

To deliver this "medicine" effectively, we need skilled technique. The absolute master of this is Teepa Snow, who developed a specific, brilliant technique called **Hand-under-Hand® (HuH)** [4].

Instead of grabbing a person's hand or arm (which the brain instantly interprets as a signal of "Control"), the HuH technique uses the anatomy of the hand to signal "Support." By sliding your hand under theirs in a comforting, palm-to-palm grasp, it gently hacks the brain's sense of where the body is in space. It makes the person feel as if they are doing the task themselves, completely bypassing the fight-or-flight response. It is the single most effective way to physically connect with a brain that has stopped processing words, offering profound comfort without triggering defensiveness.

3. Tempo: Managing the Speed of Data: A brain dealing with the loss of neural connections takes significantly longer to process incoming data. While it takes a healthy brain just milliseconds to process the command "Stand up," it can take a changing brain twenty to thirty seconds just to translate the sound into an action. This is called *synaptic lag* [5].

If you move around your parent at your normal, fast-paced speed, you are moving faster than their brain can see. You become a terrifying blur. This mismatch creates a state of *Cognitive Overload*, which often triggers severe agitation.

Instead, try to manually slow down the data transfer rate. After you ask a question or give a prompt, pause and count to ten silently in your head. Give their processing speed a chance to catch up without overheating the engine. They can no longer multitask, so a long command like *"Stand up, put on your coat, and let's go to the car"* will completely crash their system. You must break interactions down into single, manageable packets of data. If you rush the tempo, you lose the connection. *"Stand up, please."* Wait. *"Here, put on your coat."* Wait. *"Let's go to the car. Thank you."*

The Environment: Clearing the Canvas

You are learning to be the Thermostat. But even if your Tone, Touch, and Tempo are flawless, you will still struggle if the physical environment around your parent is actively attacking their Unfiltered Brain.

Remember: they receive *all* sensory input at maximum volume. What looks to you like a cozy, perfectly normal living room can look to them like a chaotic, terrifying landscape. As the brain loses its ability to filter out background data, visual clutter becomes acute anxiety. An Unfiltered Brain cannot find the spoon they need if it is hidden among a stack of mail, a newspaper, and three coffee cups on the table.

Turn off the television. Their brain can no longer separate your voice from the news anchor's voice, meaning that background noise is not neutral; it is an active, exhausting drain on their very limited processing power. You also need to increase visual contrast. A changing brain loses depth perception, meaning they need bright, even light to see where the floor ends and the wall begins. To an Unfiltered Brain, dark shadows on the floor are often misinterpreted as deep holes.

Conclusion: Be the External Regulator

Your loved one has lost their internal thermostat and can no longer regulate their own chemical state. The Paws Protocol empowers you to step in and become their *External Regulator*.

By intentionally controlling your Tone, Touch, and Tempo, you are manually lowering the temperature in the room, keeping their brain chemistry stable enough to function comfortably. You set the thermostat to a calm, loving energy, and you hold fast. It won't work perfectly every single time. But more often than not, if your thermostat holds steady, the temperature of the room will come down, and you will find your parent again in the quiet.

You have now learned the language of the Unfiltered Brain—a language spoken not in logic, but in tone, touch and tempo. It is, at its heart, the same language you have spoken for years across the living room floor with Sirius, and in the quiet morning light with Leo. You already know how to regulate a nervous system that couldn't regulate itself. You already know how to enter a frightening creature's world and make it safe. You have been practicing this all along.

13| DELIRIUM, THE AVALANCHE

Surviving the Avalanche

Imagine you are having a relatively normal week. You visited your father on Tuesday, and while he asked you the same question about the mail three times, you had a pleasant lunch. But when you get a call from his care facility on Thursday morning, the nurse tells you he is suddenly combative, heavily confused, and hallucinating that there are strangers in his room.

Or perhaps the call is different. Perhaps the nurse says, "He's just been staring at the wall for two days and won't wake up to eat."

Panic sets in. You rush over, your heart pounding, thinking: This is it. The dementia has suddenly fallen off a cliff. I have lost him.

You have not lost him, and his dementia did not suddenly plummet overnight. Brain diseases like Alzheimer's are slow, gradual fades. They do not cause a person to drop from a functioning Diamond state to a terrified, hallucinating Amber state in forty-eight hours.

What you are witnessing is not dementia. It is **Delirium**.

As the Conductor of your father's care, understanding the exact difference between these two conditions is the single most powerful tool you can carry into a hospital.

The Biology of the Crisis

If dementia is a slow, changing climate (a glacier), delirium is a sudden, violent weather event (an avalanche).

Delirium is a state of acute brain failure [1]. It is the brain's terrifying, chaotic response to an underlying *physical* crisis in the body. Because the Unfiltered Brain is already operating with frayed wiring and a vanishing chemical reserve, it has zero shock absorbers left. A physical stressor that would simply make a thirty-year-old feel "under the weather" will cause an eighty-year-old brain to completely crash.

Type 1: Hyperactive Delirium

This is the loud, explosive version. The brain goes into overdrive. The patient is restless, agitated, combative, pacing, or hallucinating. Think about our dog, Sirius. If Sirius is normally a gentle, well-behaved dog but suddenly starts pacing, snapping at you, and refusing to sleep, you don't assume he suddenly "forgot" his training. You immediately assume he stepped on a thorn, ate something toxic, or has a severe stomachache. You intuitively know that a sudden change in behavior means he is in physical pain. Your parent's Unfiltered Brain works the exact same way. They cannot say, *"My lower back hurts,"* so they translate that hidden pain into severe anxiety.

Type 2: Hypoactive Delirium

This is the "quiet" delirium. It is far more common in older adults, and far more dangerous because it is often missed. The brain doesn't explode; it shuts down. The patient becomes lethargic, stares blankly into space, sleeps all day, and withdraws completely. Think of Leo the cat. When Leo is very sick, he doesn't hiss or scratch—he hides silently under the bed and stops eating.

Hypoactive delirium is wildly underdiagnosed because it doesn't cause a disruption. In a fast-paced, overburdened medical system, a quiet patient is often assumed to be a "good" or "peaceful" patient. The doctors might look at your sleeping father and assume, *"This is just end-stage dementia."* You are the only one who knows he is actually trapped under a mental fog.

Quick Triage: Dementia vs. Delirium
- **Dementia (The Glacier):** Slow onset (months/years), generally stable attention, permanent structural change.
- **Delirium (The Avalanche):** Sudden onset (hours/days), severe fluctuations in attention, often reversible when the medical cause is treated.

Table 13.1 Quickly Triage Dementia (Glacier) vs. Delirium (Avalanche)

(Full Version can be found in Appendix 7)

All templates & forms can also be found in the **Caregiver's Toolkit**
@ www.myrxpro.com/caregivers-toolkit

The Sign	Dementia (The Glacier)	Delirium (The Avalanche)
Speed of Onset	**Slow.** Changes happen over months or years. You look back and realize they are worse than last Christmas.	**Sudden.** Changes happen over hours or days. They were fine at breakfast but confused by dinner.
Attention	**Generally Alert.** They may forget *what* you said, but they are looking at you and paying attention.	**Zoning Out.** They cannot focus. They drift off mid-sentence, look glassy-eyed, or seem "out of it."
Sleep	**Fragmented.** They might wake up at night, but they have a general routine.	**Disturbed.** They are lethargic and un-wakeable during the day, or hyper-alert and up all night.
Speech	**Word-Finding.** "Pass me the... thing." They struggle to find the right noun.	**Incoherent.** They are slurring words, speaking gibberish, or talking to people who aren't there.
The Cause	**Brain Atrophy.** A progressive structural change.	**A Medical Crisis.** Infection (UTI), Dehydration, Medication Toxicity, or Pain is causing this.
YOUR ACTION	**Use the Paws Protocol.** Use Tone, Touch, and Tempo to soothe.	**MEDICAL EMERGENCY.** This is brain failure. Call the doctor or go to the ER immediately.

The Man Who Almost Slept Through His Recovery

I received a call from a family in a state of quiet panic. Their father, Greg, an 82-year-old retired engineer with only mild memory issues, was in a top-tier rehabilitation facility following hip surgery. He was there to get stronger so he could go home.

But Greg wasn't getting stronger. He was disappearing.

"He just sleeps," his daughter told me, her voice tight with worry. "The physical therapists come, but he's too groggy to participate. They charted 'patient refused therapy.' We're ten days into a twenty-day Medicare stay, and he's barely gotten out of bed. We're terrified they're going to say he can't go home and ship him to a nursing home."

When I arrived at midday, Greg's room was dim. He was lying flat, awake but not present. He looked like a man who had given up. The staff whispered that the stress of surgery had rapidly accelerated his dementia.

I didn't buy it. Greg didn't have rapidly advancing dementia. He was suffering from Hypoactive Delirium.

This is a massive crash in GABA (regulation) and arousal systems (Histamine/Norepinephrine). The brain simply shuts down to protect itself. It is a metabolic brownout. I looked at Greg's medication chart. It was a classic recipe for brain failure.

- To help him sleep in the noisy facility, he was given a nightly dose of Tylenol PM (containing diphenhydramine, a potent anticholinergic).
- For bladder spasms, he was on another anticholinergic drug causing confusion.
- For pain, he was on a scheduled opioid that left him perpetually sedated.

He wasn't "refusing" therapy; his brain was so chemically swamped he likely couldn't process the therapist's commands. We didn't use Tone, Touch, or Tempo initially. We used deprescribing.

Working with his doctor, we immediately stopped the sleep aid and the bladder medication. We adjusted the timing of his pain meds so he wasn't at peak sedation during therapy hours.

We opened the blinds immediately to help reset his shattered circadian rhythm.

The change was startling. Two days later, his daughter called, crying in relief. *"You have to see this."*

I walked in. The blinds were open. Greg was sitting in a chair, dressed, eating lunch. His eyes were bright and focused. He knew where he was. When the therapist arrived, Greg stood up. He went home the following week.

The Efficiency of the Modern ER

When delirium strikes, your parent will likely end up in the Emergency Room. This is where your role as the Conductor of this story becomes critical, because you are stepping into a system that is not designed for this problem.

The modern ER is a miraculous, high-speed machine built to stabilize acute trauma, stop bleeding, and catch heart attacks. It is incredibly loud, blazingly bright, and moves at lightning speed. It is the absolute worst possible environment for an Unfiltered Brain experiencing sensory overload.

Because the ER is optimized for speed and safety, their immediate goal is to prevent your father from falling or pulling out an IV. If they see a confused, shouting eighty-year-old and believe this is just his "normal" dementia, they will reach for the fastest, most efficient tool in their high-volume toolkit: a chemical sedative (like a heavy antipsychotic). They are not doing this because they don't care; they are rushed professionals trying to keep a patient safe. But using a heavy sedative on a delirious brain is like putting a Band-Aid on a check-engine light. It quiets the alarm, but the engine is still on fire.

Their Baseline is the Key

This is the moment you step onto the Conductor's podium. You hold a piece of clinical data that no doctor, nurse, or medical chart possesses: **The Baseline**.

The hospital only sees a snapshot of this chaotic Thursday. You hold the entire photo album of Tuesday.

When the doctor enters, you say: "Doctor, I know he looks like he has severe dementia right now, but **this is not his baseline**. On Tuesday, he was completing a crossword puzzle and eating independently. This is an acute change. Before we use any sedatives to calm his behavior, we need to look for the underlying infection, pain, or medication issue that is causing this delirium."

By uttering the phrase *"This is not his baseline,"* you instantly change the entire trajectory of the hospital visit. You give the rushed ER doctor the structural permission they need to pause, pivot away from the psychiatric tools, and start hunting for the physical infection [2].

The Detective Work

You must redirect their attention away from the brain and toward the *body*. Delirium is almost always caused by a hidden physical trigger. Here is your investigative checklist to hand to the medical team:

- **The Usual Pharmacy Suspects:** Medications are the most common cause. Look for any new prescription or over-the-counter (OTC) drug started in the last two weeks. Watch for *Anticholinergics* (allergy meds like Benadryl, sleep aids like Tylenol PM, bladder meds),

Benzodiazepines (Xanax, Ativan), *Steroids* (Prednisone), and *Opioids.*

- **Unrecognized Infection:** A UTI in an older adult does not look like a UTI in you. They often do not have a fever, and they may not complain of burning. The only symptom might be sudden aggression or confusion [3]. Do not let a doctor dismiss a UTI because "she doesn't have a fever." Demand a urinalysis.

- **Constipation:** The gut and the brain are connected by the Vagus nerve. A severe impaction sends distress signals to the brain that manifest as agitation. Assess for "Paradoxical Diarrhea." If there is a hard rock of stool blocking the exit, liquid stool may leak around it. You might see small amounts of liquid in the diaper but feel a hard, distended belly. Do not give Imodium; you need a doctor to check for an impaction.

- **Dehydration:** The aging brain is like a sponge; when it dries out, it shrinks. Severe dehydration throws off electrolytes (like Sodium), causing neurons to misfire.

- **Sensory Deprivation:** The brain relies on eyes and ears to anchor itself in reality. If your parent is in the hospital without their glasses or hearing aids, the brain receives partial data. To fill in the gaps, it begins to hallucinate. Putting hearing aids back in is often more effective than an antipsychotic [4].

- **Unmanaged Pain:** If they have an underlying fracture from an unwitnessed fall, or severe arthritis but cannot articulate that they hurt, their brain interprets that pain signal as a threat. This leads to wild agitation. If they grimace when moved, assume pain [5].

The Protocol: Cure vs. Care

Here is the critical rule for the Conductor: You must distinguish between the *Cure* and the *Care.*

Tone, Touch, and Tempo cannot cure a urinary tract infection. You must call the doctor immediately to treat the Medical Cause (The Cure). If the doctor prescribes a sedative (Ativan/Haldol) for her agitation without running labs, you must confidently advocate: *"My mother has a vulnerable brain. A sedative will mask the symptoms of her brain failure. I want to treat the cause, not the behavior."*

While the antibiotics or IV fluids are starting to work, the brain is still crashing. *This* is where you use the Paws Protocol (The Care) to keep them safe in the chaotic ER environment:

- **Reduce Input:** Their brain is flooded with chemical noise. Ask the nurse if you can dim the harsh overhead lights in their bay. Turn off the television. Ask if you can turn down the volume on the heart monitor.

- **Remove Tethers:** Ask the staff to remove unnecessary physical tethers (like non-essential IV lines or catheters) if clinically appropriate, as these physical sensations trigger the "fight" reflex.

- **Anchor with Paws:** Use Validation ("I know you want to go home") rather than logic ("You are in the hospital") to lower the dopamine storm. Drop your tone to a low, rhythmic hum. Use the Hand-under-Hand® technique to provide deep, grounding pressure. Be the physical shield between them and the chaos of the fast machine.

The Successful Conductor

Delirium is terrifying to witness, but it is highly treatable. When the ER doctor listens to your detective work, finds the hidden UTI, and starts the antibiotics, the physical fire is put out. Within a few days, the avalanche clears. The ice melts. The hallucinations fade, the deep sleep ends, and the father you had lunch with on Tuesday returns.

You achieved this because you did not let the fast-paced system default to its quickest, heaviest pills, and you didn't let them ignore a quietly fading patient. You used your deep knowledge of his baseline to guide the medical team to the truth. You are the Conductor, and you just saved his life.

14 | THE HOSPITAL DEFENSE PLAN

Managing the Fast Machine and the Safe Discharge

The phone rings at 11:00 p.m. It is the call every care partner dreads. Barbara has fallen. The ambulance is on its way.

In this moment of panic, your instinct is to trust the hospital blindly. You assume that once she is through those sliding glass doors, she is safe.

But the modern hospital, while a miracle of trauma care, is a **hostile environment** for the geriatric brain. It is loud, bright, and disruptive. It is designed to treat acute injuries in 30-year-olds, not to protect the fragile "homeostenosis" of an 84-year-old. From the moment the ambulance doors close, Barbara is at risk of medication errors, hospital-acquired infections, and delirium.

You are the Conductor, and this is your **Hospital Defense Plan**.

Phase 1: The Hospital "Go-Bag"

You cannot effectively advocate if you are scrambling for paperwork. You need a pre-packed "Go-Bag" ready by the door. It can be small, but it is your armor; take it with you (See Figure 14.1 and Appendix 6 for the full checklist).

Stapled to the very top must be her **Master Medication**

List. Most medication errors happen in the ER simply because the doctors there don't know her history. If they don't know she takes a specific Parkinson's medication or a blood thinner, they cannot treat her safely.

Next, you need your **Ticket to Admission**—the legal and financial paperwork we discussed in Chapter 5. This includes the Medical Power of Attorney (POA), Financial POA, Living Will or POLST, her ID, and her insurance card. Accessing medical records or making rapid decisions often requires this legal standing.

Finally, remember that hospitals are sensory torture chambers. Pack her **hearing aids (with batteries or charging case) and her glasses**. This is crucial for delirium protection. If she cannot hear the doctor or see the room, her brain will fill in the gaps with hallucinations. Sensory deprivation is the fast lane to brain failure.

🍄 Pharmacist Pro Tip! 🍄

A list is great, but the actual bottles are better. When the ambulance comes, if you have time, **put all her current pill bottles into a Ziploc bag** and toss it in the Go-Bag. Why? Because lists can be outdated. The ER pharmacist can look at the date on the bottle and how many pills are left to see if she has actually been taking them. The bottle tells the true story that the list sometimes hides.

Phase 2: The Emergency Room

The ER is chaos. Your job is to be the calm, objective Medical Reporter.

Barbara may be confused by the fall or the underlying infection. If the ER doctor asks her, *"Do you have chest pain?"* and she says *"No"* because she doesn't remember, they might miss a heart attack. If she cannot remember, you must correct the answers.

This is not the time for "Validate and Reassure." Do not let her answer alone. You must provide the history: *"She has a history of AFib, she took her blood thinner this morning, and this confusion is new as of two hours ago."*

ER doctors are trained to find the simplest answer fast. They often "anchor" on a diagnosis like a UTI because it is common. If they say, *"It's just a UTI,"* but you know her symptoms are different, politely push back. *"I understand the urine looks cloudy, but her sudden inability to walk is brand new. Could we also rule out a stroke or a fracture?"*

The "Observation" Hurdle

There is a bureaucratic blind spot in the hospital system that you must actively manage: "Observation Status."

When your parent first arrives, the doctors might not be ready to officially admit them right away. Instead, they place them under "Observation" while they run tests and wait to see if the condition improves. Medically, your parent is in a hospital bed receiving care. But *bureaucratically*, they are technically considered an outpatient.

This creates a massive problem for the next phase. Medicare Part A only pays for physical rehabilitation in a Skilled Nursing Facility if the patient has had a qualifying three-day *Inpatient* hospital stay. "Observation" days do not count toward this rule.

The hospital doctors are focused on stabilizing the crisis; they are often completely unaware of how their charting affects your Medicare benefits down the line. If the hospital keeps her in Observation for three days and then tries to send her to a rehab facility, you could be hit with a devastating, unexpected out-of-pocket bill.

As the Conductor, you must track this daily. Ask the Case Manager or the floor nurse: *"Is my mother officially 'Inpatient' or is she on 'Observation' status?"* If she needs rehab but is listed as Observation, you must immediately advocate with the doctor to officially admit her so her Medicare benefits are protected.

Phase 3: Admission

If she is admitted, you are entering the most bureaucratic phase. The ER doctor does not take care of her upstairs. She will be handed off to a **Hospitalist**—an internal medicine doctor who has likely never met her and has twenty other patients.

Information gets lost in this hand-off. The Hospitalist might not know she gets anxious at night. Find the Hospitalist immediately. Hand them your Master Medication List and say, *"Hi, I know you're busy. This is Barbara. Key things to know: She has dementia, she is a high fall risk, and she gets agitated if you wake her up suddenly."* This ensures vital information doesn't get missed, and it signals that the family is an involved, prepared partner.

Phase 4: The Stay

Once she is in the bed, she faces a silent enemy: **Hospital-**

Associated Disability (HAD). Research shows that one-third of patients over seventy leave the hospital more disabled than when they arrived—not because of their illness, but because they spent days in bed.

While the hospital's goal is recovery, their workflow often defaults to keeping patients in bed to prevent falls and manage workload. We call the devices that keep them there "Tethers." An IV pole, a urinary catheter, and continuous heart monitoring function as physical restraints. They make walking so difficult that patients (and staff) give up, leading to severe muscle wasting.

Every morning, perform a **"Tether Check"** with the nurse or doctor. Ask these specific questions:

- *"Does she absolutely need continuous IV fluids, or can we switch to a 'Saline Lock' so she is free to move?"*
- *"Does she meet the criteria for the urinary catheter to come out today?"* (Catheters are a leading cause of hospital-acquired infections and a major barrier to walking).
- *"Can she walk to the bathroom with assistance?"*

Do not wait for the Physical Therapist. In a busy unit, your mother might not get walked. Ask for permission to walk her yourself (if safe): *"I am here for the next four hours. Is it safe for me to walk her in the hallway?"* Be the one who keeps her muscles working.

Figure 14.1 The Hospital "Go-Bag" Checklist, part 1

(Full Version can be found in Appendix 6)

All templates & forms can also be found in the **Caregiver's Toolkit** @ www.myrxpro.com/caregivers-toolkit

Instructions: Photocopy this page, or download a copy from MyRxPro.com. Pack the items listed below into a brightly colored tote bag and keep it by your front door. When the ambulance is called, you do not have time to think. Grab this bag.

The Critical Documents

These are your "Ticket to Entry" and your "Shield."

◯ **Master Medication List:** Two copies (one for the ER doctor, one for the nurse).
Tip: Put all current pill bottles into a Ziploc bag and throw them in, too.

◯ **Medical Power of Attorney (MPOA):** A photocopy of your Medical POA. (Sometimes called a HCPOA)

◯ **Financial Power of Attorney / Durable Power of Attorney:** A photocopy of your Financial POA.
(Sometimes just called the POA)

◯ **Living will / POLST Form:** Living will are resuscitation wishes of your parent. POLST is the pink or green
form are physician order dictating resuscitation orders.

◯ **ID & Insurance Cards:** Photocopies of the front and back of her insurance/Medicare cards and photo ID.

Figure 14.2 The Hospital "Go-Bag" Checklist, part 2

(Full Version can be found in Appendix 6)

All templates & forms can also be found in the **Caregiver's Toolkit**
@ www.myrxpro.com/caregivers-toolkit

The Sensory Kit

Hospitals are sensory deprivation chambers. Protect her input channels to prevent delirium.

○ Hearing Aids: Plus extra batteries and the charger.
○ Glasses: In a hard case labeled with her name.
○ Dentures: Plus a labeled denture cup and adhesive.

Comfort & Anchors

Humanize them to the staff and soothe her amygdala.

○ One Familiar Item: A small fleece blanket or a shawl that reminds them of home.
○ One Family Photo: Tape this to the wall or bed rail. It gives your loved one an anchor to who they are and It reminds busy staff that this patient is a person who is loved.
○ Phone Charger: For your phone. It's going to be a long night.

The "STOP" Sign

Write the following on a bright Neon Index Card and tape it to the top of the Medication List.

ATTENTION: SENSITIVE BRAIN Patient has a history of Cognitive Decline.

1. NO Benadryl (Diphenhydramine)

2. NO Benzodiazepines (Ativan/Xanax) These medications cause immediate Delirium/Agitation for this patient.

If Agitated: Please call family/POA first to assist with calming.

Protecting the Unfiltered Brain

Nighttime is when the Unfiltered Brain crashes. If Barbara becomes confused and yells, the standard hospital protocol is often a chemical sedative (like Ativan or Benadryl).

These drugs are rocket fuel for delirium. They can turn a temporary confusion into a permanent cognitive decline. Tape a note above her bed and tell the Charge Nurse: *"My mother has a sensitive brain. Please, NO Benadryl and NO Benzodiazepines for sleep or anxiety. If she gets agitated, call me first."*

Phase 5: The Discharge

Modern hospitals function as high-efficiency stabilization centers. Because their primary goal is to treat acute crises and make room for the next emergency, they may try to discharge Barbara the moment her vital signs are stable, which is often before she is functionally ready to go home.

If they say, *"She is going home tomorrow,"* but you know she cannot walk to the bathroom or get out of bed safely, do not passively accept the discharge. Use your Conductor's voice: *"I cannot accept this discharge. It is an Unsafe Discharge. She cannot perform her ADLs (Activities of Daily Living) and I am not trained to lift her. We need to prioritize Safety over Speed."*

If the Case Manager denies this request, say these exact words: *"I am formally requesting the Important Message from Medicare form to file an immediate appeal with the QIO (Quality Improvement Organization)."* This is your federally protected legal right, and it legally stops the discharge clock.

Finally, the **Medication Reconciliation** is where the most dangerous errors happen. The hospital doctor might have stopped her thyroid pill during the crisis or doubled her blood pressure pill and forgotten to switch it back. Do not leave the building until you compare the hospital's Discharge Med List against your Master Med List. Ask: *"Why is she on two blood pressure pills now? Did you mean to restart her thyroid med?"*

Conclusion: You Are Armed

The hospital is a powerful system designed for speed and efficiency. It is not designed for the slow, complex needs of an eighty-four-year-old.

By knowing the rules—packing the Go-Bag, avoiding the Observation Trap, performing the Tether Check, and executing the Discharge Appeal—you turn the odds in Barbara's favor. You act as the shield that protects her from the fast machine, ensuring she has the time and safety she actually needs to heal.

15 | THE NURSING HOME QUESTION

A Compassionate Checklist for When 'At Home' Is No Longer Safe

There is a question that haunts the quiet, 3:00 a.m. thoughts of so many care partners. It's a question steeped in love, guilt, exhaustion, and a deep-seated fear of breaking a sacred promise.

You may have even said the words aloud to your mother, years ago: *"Mom, don't you ever worry. I will never put you in a nursing home."*

At the time, you meant it with every fiber of your being. It felt like the ultimate declaration of love and loyalty. But you said it before you truly understood the biological changes ahead. You said it before the nights of fractured sleep, before the constant worry about falls, before the two-a.m. phone calls when she was disoriented and scared, and before the physical and emotional toll of round-the-clock care started to erode your own health, your career, and your relationships.

Now, you find yourself at a breaking point. Your mother, Barbara, is now unsafe to be left alone, even for an hour. Her needs have surpassed what you can physically and emotionally provide within the four walls of her home or your own. The idea of "a home" has been simmering in the back of your mind, a thought so filled with guilt that you can barely let it surface. It feels like you are contemplating a failure, an admission of defeat, a betrayal of your most solemn vow.

Let this chapter be your guide to meet you in that dark, quiet, 3:00 a.m. place. Its purpose is to completely reframe this impossible decision.

I want to help you see that considering a move to a higher level of care—whether it's assisted living, memory care, or a skilled nursing facility—is not an act of abandonment. In many circumstances, it is the most loving, responsible, and courageous act a care partner can perform. It is a decision that prioritizes your parent's safety and your own survival.

Safety Over Location

Before we get to the checklist, we must revisit our core philosophy from Chapter 2: *Function Over Numbers*. When it comes to long-term care, we must expand that to **Safety and Quality of Life Over Location**.

Our society has created a powerful narrative that "aging in place" at home is the ultimate, gold-standard goal. And for many people, for a very long time, it absolutely is. But there comes a point for some individuals where the location of "home" begins to actively work against the goal of safety and well-being.

There is nothing loving or noble about a parent "aging in place" if that place involves them being socially isolated, at high risk for a catastrophic fall, receiving inadequate nutrition, and being cared for by a care partner who is themselves collapsing under the strain. At that point, "home" has become a place of risk, rather than a place of sanctuary.

The true goal is not to keep them in a specific building. The true goal is to ensure they are in an environment where they are as safe, engaged, comfortable, and as well-cared for as possible. Sometimes, the place that can best deliver that high-quality, 24/7 care is not a private residence, but a community designed specifically for that purpose.

This shift in thinking—from location to quality of life—is the first step in releasing yourself from the guilt of that long-ago promise. You are not breaking your promise to care for them; you are evolving it to meet their changing biology.

A Lesson in Loving Detachment

Last year, your wonderful dog, Sirius, had to have surgery on his knee. The recovery was difficult. For the first two weeks, he couldn't put any weight on his back leg. As a 90-pound golden retriever, he was too heavy for you to safely carry up and down the back steps to the yard by yourself.

You tried for a day, struggling and straining, nearly dropping him twice. You were terrified you would hurt him or yourself. You quickly realized your "at-home" setup was inadequate for his post-operative needs.

Did you love him any less for this realization? Of course not. In fact, your love compelled you to seek a better solution. Perhaps you borrowed a special sling-harness from a friend that allowed you to safely support his weight. You changed his "environment" so he slept downstairs to avoid the steps entirely. And if his needs had been even greater, you would have considered a temporary stay at a veterinary rehabilitation facility where professionals could have cared for him with the right equipment and 24/7 expertise.

The goal was never to stubbornly "do it all yourself" at home. The goal was to ensure Sirius had the safest and most effective recovery possible. Your love for him demanded that you recognize your own limitations and seek expert help.

It is the exact same principle for Barbara. Your love for her must include the wisdom to recognize when her needs require a level of safety and skilled care that you, as one person, can no longer provide at home.

The Conductor's Checklist: An Objective Assessment

Making this decision from a place of crisis is agonizing. Making it from a place of clear-eyed, compassionate assessment is empowering. To do that, we need a tool.

This checklist is a tool for self-reflection and honest assessment. Go through the template provided in Appendix 4 with a pen and paper. Be brutally honest. There are no right or wrong answers, only clarity. A single "yes" may not mean it's time, but a cascade of them is a powerful signal that the current situation is no longer sustainable.

Part 1: Assessing Your Parent's Needs and Safety

- **Falls:** Has your parent fallen more than once in the last six months? Are you in a constant state of anxiety about them falling when you are not there? Do they have bruises they can't explain?
- **Wandering & Environmental Safety:** Has your parent ever wandered out of the house and gotten lost, even for a few minutes? Have you found a stovetop burner left on or the front door left unlocked and open?
- **Activities of Daily Living (ADLs):** Is your parent now consistently unable to perform two or more of the core

ADLs without significant hands-on help: bathing, dressing, grooming, eating, getting to and from the toilet, or moving from a bed to a chair?

- **Medical & Medication Complexity:** Is their medication schedule so complex that you are terrified of making a mistake? Do they have a medical condition (like needing regular injections, wound care, or oxygen) that requires skilled care you are not trained to provide?

- **Behavioral Challenges:** If they have dementia, are their behavioral symptoms (like aggression, paranoia, or severe sundowning) becoming more than you can safely manage? Are they a potential danger to themselves or to you?

🐾 Professor's Facts! 🐾

A "Lone Wolf" is a romantic concept in movies, but in biology, it is a tragedy. A wolf separated from the pack has elevated cortisol (stress) levels and a significantly shorter lifespan. They are social obligates—they require connection to survive.

Just like Sirius and his ancestors, we humans are social beings, which explains why social isolation is detrimental to our health.

- **Social Isolation:** Is your parent spending most of their day alone, with little to no social interaction beyond your visits? Have they lost connection with friends and hobbies because it's too difficult for them to participate?

- **Home Environment:** Is the house itself no longer safe? Is it a multi-story home that requires them to navigate stairs? Is the bathroom too small to accommodate a walker or wheelchair? Is the home cluttered and a significant trip hazard?

Figure 15.1 Aging in Place Safety Assessment, part 1 (first)

(Full Version can be found in Appendix 4)

All templates & forms can also be found in the **Caregiver's Toolkit @ www.myrxpro.com/caregivers-toolkit**

This tool is designed to help you make an objective, data-driven assessment of whether "aging in place" is still the safest option for your parent—and for you.

Part 1: Assessing Your Parent's Needs and Safety
Focus on the reality of the last 6 months.

Falls: Has your parent fallen more than once in the last six months? Are you in a constant state of anxiety about them falling when you are not there? Do they have bruises they can't explain?

Wandering & Safety: Has your parent ever wandered out of the house and gotten lost? Have you found a stovetop burner left on or the front door left unlocked and open?

Activities of Daily Living (ADLs): Is your parent consistently unable to perform **two or more** of these core tasks without hands-on help?

○ *Bathing*	○ *Grooming*	○ *Toileting*
○ *Dressing*	○ *Eating*	○ *Transferring*

Figure 15.2 Aging in Place Safety Assessment, part 1 (second)

(Full Version can be found in Appendix 4)

All templates & forms can also be found in the **Caregiver's Toolkit** @ **www.myrxpro.com/caregivers-toolkit**

○ **Medical Complexity:** Is their medication schedule so complex that you are terrified of making a mistake? Do they require skilled care (injections, wound care, oxygen) you are not trained to provide?

○ **Behavioral Challenges:** If they have dementia, are symptoms like aggression, paranoia, or severe sundowning becoming more than you can safely manage? Are they a danger to themselves or you?

○ **Social Isolation:** Is your parent spending most of their day alone with little interaction beyond your visits? Have they lost connection with friends because it is too difficult to participate?

○ **Home Environment:** Is the house itself unsafe? (e.g., Multi-story with stairs, bathroom too small for a walker, significant clutter/trip hazards).

Part 2: Assessing Your Own Well-being and Breaking Point

This is the part we often ignore, but it is just as important. Your well-being is not a selfish luxury; it is the cornerstone of your ability to provide loving care. You cannot pour from an empty cup, and you cannot conduct an orchestra if you are collapsing on the podium.

- **Your Physical Health:** Are you chronically sleep-deprived? Have you been ignoring your own medical appointments or health issues because you have no time? Has the physical strain of lifting or transferring your parent caused you injury?

- **Your Mental Health:** Do you feel a constant sense of dread, anxiety, or resentment? Are you showing signs of clinical depression? Have you lost interest in the activities and relationships that used to bring you joy?

- **Your "Why":** Be honest with yourself. Are you continuing to provide care at home out of a genuine belief that it is the best possible situation, or are you doing it primarily out of guilt, fear of judgment, or a broken promise?

- **Your Support System:** Are you the sole care partner with little to no regular help from other family members? Do you feel completely and utterly alone in this responsibility?

- **Your Other Responsibilities:** Is your career suffering? Are your relationships with your spouse or your own children becoming strained to the breaking point because your care partner role consumes all of your available time and emotional energy?

Take a long, hard look at your answers. If you have checked multiple boxes, particularly in both sections, that is not a sign of your failure. It is a sign that the needs of the situation have grown larger than the resources available in the home environment. It is a clear, data-driven signal that it is time to at least explore other options.

Figure 15.3 Aging in Place Safety Assessment, part 2

(Full Version can be found in Appendix 4)

All templates & forms can also be found in the **Caregiver's Toolkit** @ **www.myrxpro.com/caregivers-toolkit**

Part 2: Assessing Your Own Well-Being

You cannot pour from an empty cup.
These questions are just as important as Part 1.

- ○ **Your Physical Health:** Are you chronically sleep-deprived? Have you ignored your own medical appointments? Has lifting or moving your parent caused you physical injury?

- ○ **Your Mental Health:** Do you feel constant dread, anxiety, or resentment? are you showing signs of depression or loss of interest in things that used to bring you joy?

- ○ **Your "Why":** Are you providing care at home primarily out of guilt, fear of judgment, or a promise made years ago before you understood the reality?

- ○ **Your Support System:** Are you the sole care partner with little to no regular help? Do you feel completely alone in this responsibility?

- ○ **Your Other Responsibilities:** Is your career suffering? Are your relationships with your spouse or children straining to the breaking point?

Conclusion: An Act of Love, Not Abandonment

The decision to move a parent to a long-term care facility is one of the most painful a child can make. But it does not have to be a tragedy. When made for the right reasons—for safety, for appropriate medical care, for social engagement, and for the preservation of your own health—it is a decision that can bring peace, security, and a new kind of quality of life to everyone involved.

Moving your parent to a good care community does not mean you are stopping your care partnership journey. It means your role is changing. You are released from the exhausting, 24/7 duties of a hands-on nurse, cook, and housekeeper.

You are freed to return to your primary, most important role: that of a loving, engaged, and rested son or daughter. You can now visit your mother not to change her linens or administer medication, but to sit with her, hold her hand, share a story, and simply enjoy her company. You get to be her child again.

In many ways, this choice is the ultimate fulfillment of your promise to care for her. It is the brave, responsible, and profoundly loving act of admitting that the best possible care is no longer something you can provide alone. It is ensuring she gets the safety and support she needs, even when it breaks your heart to do it.

How to Manage the Facility from the Inside

You have made the difficult decision. Barbara has moved into a Care Home. This was an act of love to ensure her safety. But your job is not done. Because facilities must prioritize routine and efficiency to manage dozens of residents, your goal is to ensure Barbara's individual needs don't get lost in the shuffle.

Tool 1: The "Pop-In" Strategy

Facilities put on a show for scheduled tours. To know the truth, you must visit when the "Management" is gone. Visit during the evening "sundown" hours or on weekends.

The "Sensory" Check: Is the environment chaotic? Are televisions blaring news programs that trigger anxiety?

The "Care" Check: Are residents being helped to eat, or are trays left untouched?

Tool 2: The Staffing Ratio Audit

While specific ratios vary by state, systemic understaffing is a known issue across long-term care. You need to verify if there are enough humans to safely care for the residents. The night shift is often where facilities run the leanest. Administrative models often assume residents are sleeping, but the reality is that residents with dementia frequently experience sundowning, wandering, and require nighttime toileting. If the ratio is 1 to 30, that means one CNA has just two minutes per hour for your mother. This is why "incontinence" suddenly appears in nursing homes—not because the bladder failed, but because the staffing was too lean.

When you ask the question, use this script to signal you know the difference between "scheduled" and "actual."

"I know staffing can fluctuate, but what is your typical actual CNA-to-resident ratio on the night shift? And does that count 'all hands' or just the floor staff actively assigned to resident care?"

The Red Flag Answer: "We staff according to census and acuity." (This is a non-answer).

The Green Flag Answer: "We try to keep it at 1 to 12 or 1 to 15 at night." This is what is required by 2024 CMS Federal requirements.

Tool 3: The "Chemical Restraint" Check

When a facility is understaffed, they cannot spend time using the Paws Protocol (Tone, Touch, Tempo) to calm an agitated resident. It is faster to give them a pill.

Antipsychotics are frequently used off-label to sedate dementia patients. This is **Chemical Restraint**.

These drugs cause toxic stress on a brain already in failure. They can lead to accelerated cognitive decline and permanent damage.

Once a month, request her **Medication Administration Record (MAR)** and audit it. Look for new prescriptions you didn't approve. *"I see Mom was started on an antipsychotic. I* *did not authorize this. These drugs carry more risk than benefit. I want to see documentation of what non-drug interventions were tried first, and we need to taper this off immediately."*

Tool 4: The Care Plan Meeting

Every quarter, the facility should hold a "Care Plan Meeting." Come with an agenda.

Weight & Nutrition: Is she losing weight? Is she having difficulty chewing or swallowing?

Mobility: Is she participating in activities, or is she becoming bedbound due to chemical sedation?

Social: Is she isolated? Social isolation is a key indicator that the current situation may not be sustainable.

Figure 16.1 The Transition Day Checklist, part 1

(Full Version can be found in Appendix 9)

All templates & forms can also be found in the **Caregiver's Toolkit** @ **www.myrxpro.com/caregivers-toolkit**

Part 1: The "Face Sheet" (Bring 3 Copies)

Do not rely on the hospital to send the records. Systems fail. You are the courier. Create a single-page document with the following information in large, bold type. Hand one copy to the **Director of Nursing**, one to the **Unit Manager**, and tape one to the **wall inside the room** (if allowed).

- **Patient Name & Preferred Name:** (e.g., "Barbara Smith, prefers 'Barb'")
- **Primary Contact:** Your Name & Cell Phone Number.
- **Code Status:** (DNR / DNI / Full Code) — *Attach a copy of the POLST/MOLST form.*

- **The "Big Three" Alerts:**
    - ○ Fall Risk (e.g., "Tries to get up without help at night")
    - ○ Swallowing/Choking Risk (e.g., "Needs thickened liquids")
    - ○ Allergies (e.g., "Penicillin," "Latex")

- **Current Medication List:** A clean list of what she is actually taking.

- **Baseline Status:** A one-sentence description of her "Normal." (e.g., *"Barb is usually confused in the mornings but clear in the evenings. She can feed herself but needs help cutting meat."*)

Figure 16.2 The Transition Day Checklist, part 2

(Full Version can be found in Appendix 9)

All templates & forms can also be found in the **Caregiver's Toolkit**
@ **www.myrxpro.com/caregivers-toolkit**

Part 2: The Room Sweep (Safety Check)
Perform this check immediately upon entering the room.
Do not unpack until these are verified.

The Bed:
- ◯ Is the bed at the lowest possible height setting?
- ◯ Are the brakes locked on the bed wheels?
- ◯ Is the mattress firm/stable?

The Path:
- ◯ Is the path from the bed to the bathroom clear of cords, rugs, or furniture?
- ◯ Is the floor dry and non-slip?

The Equipment:
- ◯ **Call Light:** Is it plugged in? Does it work? Is it clipped within reach of the pillow?
- ◯ **Assist Bars:** Are the grab bars in the bathroom secure (give them a hard shake)?
- ◯ **Oxygen/Suction:** (If applicable) Are the lines connected and flowing?

Figure 16.3 The Transition Day Checklist, part 3

(Full Version can be found in Appendix 9)

All templates & forms can also be found in the **Caregiver's Toolkit** @ www.myrxpro.com/caregivers-toolkit

Part 4: The "Paws" (Comfort Anchors)
The goal is to reduce cortisol (stress) to prevent delirium.

- ◯ **Scent/Touch:** A familiar pillow with a bright, recognizable pillowcase.

- ◯ **Visual:** A large photo of family or pets placed where she can see it from the bed.

- ◯ **Auditory:** Noise-canceling headphones or a white noise machine if the hallway is loud.

- ◯ **The "Go-Bag" Transfer:** Ensure her glasses, hearing aids (with batteries), and dentures are in the room and labeled with her name.

Part 5: The Exit Protocol
- ◯ Confirm the staff knows you are leaving.
- ◯ Ensure the Call Light is in your parent's hand.
- ◯ Say goodbye. (Keep it brief to minimize agitation).
- ◯ **Go home and sleep.**

The Hardest Day: The Transition Protocol

The day you move Barbara is not just a logistical challenge; it is a sensory shock. The smell of industrial cleaner, the sound of call bells, the sight of strangers. This checklist is your way of imposing order on that sensory chaos.

We have talked about the metrics and the staffing ratios. But we need to pause and talk about the actual day. Moving a parent into a facility—whether it is Assisted Living or a Skilled Nursing Facility—is one of the most emotionally brutal days you will experience as a care partner.

You will feel guilty. You will feel relieved. And then you will feel guilty about being relieved. This is normal.

But while your heart is breaking, you have a lot of work to prepare. The facility is most vulnerable to errors in the first 48 hours. The staff doesn't know Barbara yet. They don't know that she hides her pills or that she falls when she tries to use the toilet at night.

Here is your **Transition Day Checklist** to ensure the transition goes smoothly:

The "Face Sheet" Handoff: Do not rely on the hospital to send the records. Bring a printed "Face Sheet" (one page) containing: Her Full Diagnosis List, Her Current Med List (Double-checked by you), and **Three Critical Alerts** (e.g., "High Fall Risk," "Allergic to Penicillin," "Deaf in Left Ear"). Hand this to the Director of Nursing.

The Room Sweep: Before you unpack a single bag, check the room. Is the call light within reach? Is the bed at the lowest setting? Is there a clear path to the bathroom? If the room feels unsafe, do not leave her alone in it.

The "Comfort Anchor": In the sterile environment of a facility, Barbara needs a scent or a texture that signals "Safety." Bring her own pillow (brightly colored case so it doesn't get lost in laundry). Bring a photo of the dog. These are not just sentimental; they are biological signals that lower cortisol and reduce the risk of "delirium" (sudden confusion).

Establish the "Point Person": Do not leave until you have the name and direct phone number of the Unit Manager. Say: "I know you are busy. I want to be a partner, not a pest. If I see something wrong, who is the specific person I should call?"

By managing the logistics of the Transition Day, you buy yourself the emotional space to handle the grief.

Conclusion

There is a final, heavy emotion we must address before we close this chapter: **The Drop-Off Guilt.**

When you drive away from the facility that first night, leaving Barbara in a strange bed with strange sounds, you will likely feel a crushing sense of failure. You will feel like you have broken a promise to keep her safe in her own home.

Let me try to reframe this for you.

You have not abandoned her. You have outsourced the heavy lifting.

By moving Barbara to a facility, you are acknowledging a physical reality: The level of care she needs has exceeded what one human being can provide in a living room. You are hiring a team to handle the hard work—the lifting, the washing, the dispensing of pills.

But you are not resigning from your role. You are simply changing your position on the podium.

Before, you were playing all the roles—nurse, cook, cleaner, safety officer.

Now, you are purely the **Conductor**.

Your job now is not to lift her; it is to watch the people who do. Your job is to be the "Pop-In" that keeps the staff alert. Your job is to bring the specific knowledge of who she is into this sterile building so that the system sees a *person*, not a *bed number*.

This move also gives you something precious back: **The**

permission to rest.

Because you are no longer exhausted by the 3:00 AM fall or the 6:00 AM laundry, you can use your limited energy for connection. You can sit by her bed and hold her hand without mentally calculating when her next diaper change is due. You can go back to being a daughter, a son, or a partner, rather than just a tired caregiver.

The facility provides the walls. You provide the advocacy. The facility provides the metrics. You provide the love.

Barbara is in a new building now. But you are still the Conductor who ensures she is safe. Go home. Sleep. The Conductor needs to be rested for the next shift.

PART 5 | THE PROFESSORS

The Pawsitive Prescription

We have come a long way. We have audited medicine cabinets, mastered the 8-minute appointment, and navigated some of the most difficult conversations a care partner will ever have. You have been given systems, scripts, and checklists—the hard, practical tools of the "Conductor's Toolkit." You now have the skills to manage the most challenging aspects of your parent's care.

Now, we turn to the heart.

The final two chapters of this book are dedicated to your most unexpected and arguably most effective therapeutic therapy: your senior cat and dog. This is not just a collection of heartwarming anecdotes. This is a serious look at the science of the human-animal bond and, more importantly, a deep dive into the practical, clinical skills that caring for an aging animal teaches us.

Sirius and Leo are more than companions; they are your resident professors of non-verbal communication, your Zen masters of living in the moment, and your daily prescription for de-stressing a weary soul. It is through them that we will learn the final, most profound lessons on our journey to becoming confident, compassionate care partners.

It is time for the Pawsitive Prescription.

17| Lessons in Appetite and Agency from the Finicky Cat

A Masterclass in Observation

Your sixteen-year-old cat, Leo, has always been a creature of impeccable routine. Breakfast at 7:01 a.m., a post-meal grooming session on the sunlit patch of rug, a four-hour nap on your favorite armchair, followed by a brief tour of the perimeter before his second nap. His life has been a testament to the comforting power of predictability.

But for the past week, something has been off. The change is subtle, almost imperceptible. He no longer cleans his food bowl with his usual surgical precision; he eats half and walks away. He made the leap to the back of the sofa yesterday, but there was a moment's hesitation you'd never seen before. He just seems more... quiet. More withdrawn.

Your first thought is, "He's just getting old." It's an easy and comforting dismissal. But the skilled care partner, the one you are becoming, knows better. You know that in a creature who cannot speak, **behavior is data.** A subtle change is often the first and only clue to a significant underlying problem. Your cat is not being "finicky"; he is trying to tell you something is wrong. He is communicating in the only language he has.

This chapter is about learning to listen to that language. The challenge of decoding the silent signals of a stoic animal is a masterclass in the single most important skill required to care for a non-communicative human being, whether it's a parent in the advanced stages of dementia or one recovering from a debilitating stroke. It is the art and science of keen, non-judgmental observation.

The Science of the Stoic: Understanding Feline Cognitive Dysfunction

Just as humans and dogs can develop age-related dementia, so too can cats. The condition, known as **Feline Cognitive Dysfunction (FCD)**, is a real, progressive, neurological disease. It is far less studied and likely underdiagnosed because of a cat's innate ability to hide vulnerability—a survival instinct held over from their wild ancestors [1]. A cat showing obvious signs of illness was an easy target for a larger predator. Your Leo carries that ancient legacy of stoicism.

While research is ongoing, the underlying pathology of FCD is thought to be similar to what we see in humans and dogs: a buildup of those now-familiar beta-amyloid plaques between nerve cells, along with other age-related changes like oxidative stress and chronic inflammation that lead to the death of neurons. This brain damage can manifest in a collection of symptoms that veterinary behaviorists often summarize with the acronym **VISHDAAL** [2]:

Vocalization: Increased or unusual howling, especially at night.

Interaction changes: Becoming unusually clingy or, more commonly, withdrawn and irritable.

Sleep/Wake cycle changes: Pacing at night, sleeping more during the day.

House soiling: Inappropriate urination or defecation outside the litter box.

Disorientation: Getting lost in familiar places, staring blankly at walls.

Activity changes: Apathy, loss of interest in play, or aimless pacing.

Anxiety/Learning & Memory deficits: Forgetting routines, increased fearfulness.

Seeing these symptoms described in a clinical context for a cat can be incredibly illuminating. It reframes them from frustrating behaviors into neurological symptoms. When Leo stares at a wall, we can now see it not as a bizarre quirk, but as a potential sign of disorientation. This scientific lens helps us approach Barbara's similar behaviors with more compassion and less fear.

Decoding the Data: What Could Be Wrong with Leo?

Your core observation that Leo is "off his food" and more withdrawn is your starting point. A less experienced care companion might simply change his food brand, assuming he has become a "picky eater." But you know this is a clinical sign that requires a differential diagnosis—a list of possible underlying causes. Your job is to gather more data for the veterinarian. Here are the most common ailments of an older cat that present with just these subtle signs:

Dental Disease: This is an incredibly common, painful, and frequently missed condition in senior cats. The cat's instinct is to hide this oral pain. He may be hungry, but the act of chewing is agonizing, so he gives up and walks away. Watch him eat. Is he dropping food from his mouth? Does he chew only on one side? Is there a new or worsening odor on his breath? Does he flinch if you gently touch his cheek?

Chronic Kidney Disease (CKD): As we learned in Chapter 3, a cat's hyper-efficient kidneys are their evolutionary superpower and their biological Achilles' heel. CKD is an epidemic in senior cats, affecting an estimated 30-50% of cats over the age of 15. One of the first and most common signs is nausea and a resulting loss of appetite. The litter box is your data hub. Is he urinating more frequently? Are the urine clumps in the litter larger than usual? This indicates his kidneys can no longer concentrate urine effectively. Is he spending more time at the water bowl?

Osteoarthritis: The chronic pain from degenerative joint disease is another deeply underdiagnosed condition in cats. They don't limp like dogs. Instead, they demonstrate pain through a change in behavior. A landmark paper on this topic revealed how subtle these signs are [3]. The hesitation you saw before he jumped is a critical piece of data. Has he stopped sleeping on a high perch he used to love? Is he more hesitant to use the stairs? Is his coat looking unkempt or matted, particularly over his lower back? This can happen because it has become too painful for him to twist and groom himself properly.

Hyperthyroidism: Another common ailment of older cats, where the thyroid gland goes into overdrive, creating a hyper-metabolic state. This can cause a strange combination of a ravenous appetite but with progressive weight loss. It can also cause vomiting, increased thirst, and restlessness, which can look like the vocalization and anxiety of FCD.

You see the pattern. A single, subtle behavioral change—"eating less"—can be a sign of a mouth problem, a kidney problem, a joint problem, or a hormonal problem. Without careful observation, the root cause is unknowable.

The Lesson for Barbara: Applying the "Leo Framework"

This process of careful, multi-faceted observation is the greatest skill Leo can teach you. It is a framework you can apply directly to caring for a non-communicative Barbara. When a parent with advanced dementia stops eating or becomes more agitated, the cause is very often not "just the dementia." It is a physical problem they can no longer articulate. Your job is to become the same keen observer for her that you are for your cat.

Scenario 1: She refuses to eat. The **Leo Framework** tells you to resist the simple explanation and dig deeper. You go through your differential diagnosis.

Is it her mouth? Ask her if her teeth hurt. Look for grimacing when she chews or her pocketing food in one cheek to avoid a painful spot. Poorly fitting dentures are a common culprit.

Could it be nausea? Has she started a new medication (like a cholinesterase inhibitor or an antibiotic) known to cause nausea? Look for other subtle signs like restlessness, burping, or swallowing repeatedly.

Is it her joints? Is the chair she's sitting in at the dining table too low and painful to sit in for long? Perhaps eating on the sofa where she is more comfortable would be a better option.

Could it be constipation? A severely backed-up gut is a very common cause of appetite loss in older adults.

Scenario 2: She cries out or becomes agitated, especially when you help her change or move. The "Leo Framework" teaches you to assume pain first.

One of the great tragedies of dementia care is undiagnosed and untreated pain. Your parent may not be able to say, "My back hurts when you move my legs that way." They express that pain through what looks like aggression or resistance—a cry, a swatting hand, a grimace.

Become a student of her non-verbal cues. Where do you see her wince? Does she guard one part of her body? Does she resist when you try to lift one arm to put on her sleeve? This is invaluable data to bring to her doctor. Often, a simple, scheduled dose of acetaminophen before you help her with her morning care can transform the entire experience for both of you.

Scenario 3: She begins having "accidents" and is newly incontinent. The Leo Framework asks you to look for a root cause beyond "old age."

The #1 cause of new-onset incontinence in an older adult is a **urinary tract infection (UTI)**. It can also cause the confusion and agitation of delirium. Before assuming this is a permanent decline, you must rule out a treatable infection.

What are the logistics? Can she physically get to the bathroom fast enough? Is the path cluttered? Does she have arthritis in her hands that makes unbuttoning her pants difficult? Simple environmental changes or different clothing can sometimes solve the problem.

Leo, in his quiet, stoic mystery, forces you to become a better clinician. He teaches you to trust your observations, to look for patterns, to generate a list of possibilities, and to always assume that a change in behavior is a communication. It is a message that something is wrong. This skill is how you protect those who can no longer articulate their needs. It is how you become their most powerful and compassionate advocate.

18| Lessons in Mobility and Joy from the
Good Old Dog

A Masterclass in Comfort and a Prescription for Your Own Health

You've had a brutal day. You spent two hours on the phone fighting with an insurance company about a denied claim for Barbara's medication. You then had a tense, circular conversation with your mother, who was agitated and confused. You are emotionally drained, your reserves of patience have run dry, and you feel the familiar, heavy cloak of being a care partner settling over you. You walk in your front door, collapse onto the couch, and put your head in your hands.

A moment later, you feel a gentle, wet nose nudge your elbow. Your eleven-year-old dog, Sirius, rests his heavy, graying head on your lap and looks up at you with those deep, soulful eyes. He doesn't offer advice. He doesn't ask you to do anything. He is simply *present*. You begin to stroke his soft ears, and as you do, you feel your heart rate begin to slow. Your breathing deepens. The knot of tension in your shoulders starts to release.

In that simple, wordless interaction, you have just received the most powerful medicine available for a stressed-out human soul.

This chapter is about the science of that medicine. While Leo the cat teaches us the critical clinical skill of observation, your dog Sirius teaches you the equally important therapeutic skill of providing uncomplicated comfort. And in doing so, he offers a powerful prescription for healing your own weary heart.

The Science of Comfort: How Sirius Hacks Your Brain

The profound sense of calm you feel when petting Sirius is not your imagination. It is a well-documented cascade of powerful neurochemical events, a testament to the co-evolution of humans and dogs over tens of thousands of years.

The gentle, rhythmic act of petting a friendly, familiar dog triggers the release of **oxytocin** in your brain [1]. This neurochemical is often called the "love hormone" or "bonding hormone," the same one that floods a new mother's brain to foster feelings of connection and well-being. Oxytocin is a powerful anti-stress agent; it actively lowers levels of the stress hormone cortisol, can reduce blood pressure, and promotes feelings of calm and social trust. When you interact with your dog, you are giving yourself a dose of biological anti-anxiety agent.

What is truly beautiful is that this is a two-way street. Studies measuring oxytocin levels have shown that the dog's brain *also* releases this hormone when being petted by a beloved human. It's a shared, physiological experience of comfort that creates a positive biochemical feedback loop of mutual affection and stress reduction. You are not just calming yourself; you are participating in a scientifically-validated, cross-species wellness program.

Human relationships are complex. Caring for a parent with dementia is a tangled web of past history, present challenges, and future fears. The beauty of your relationship with Sirius is its stunning simplicity. You provide him with food, a walk, and affection. In return, he gives you unconditional love and gratitude. There is no subtext, no hidden resentment, no unresolved conflict. The feedback is clean, immediate, and always positive. This provides an essential emotional "reset" from the exhausting complexity of human care partnerships. For the Overloaded Brain, this simplicity is not a luxury; it is a vital respite.

The Science of Relief: New Hope for Your Aching Dog

Just as Sirius provides you with comfort, your role is also to provide comfort for him. This, too, offers a profound lesson. Watching him struggle with his own arthritis pain teaches us about modern, multi-modal approaches to pain management that go far beyond just a pill and can inform how we think about care for Barbara.

For years, your main tool for Sirius's arthritis was likely a daily chewable NSAID prescribed by your vet. While effective, you probably also worried about the potential long-term side effects on his liver or stomach. But the world of veterinary pain management has made incredible strides, moving toward more targeted and safer long-term solutions.

The New Injection Monoclonal Antibodies: This is one of the most exciting breakthroughs in modern veterinary medicine. There are now once-a-month injections available for dogs (**Librela**™ (bedinvetmab)) and for cats (**Solensia**™, (frunevetmab)) that specifically target osteoarthritis pain. These are not traditional drugs or steroids. They are monoclonal antibodies—highly specific, engineered proteins that are designed to do one job with extreme precision [2, 3].

A key molecule responsible for amplifying and transmitting chronic arthritis pain signals in the body is a protein called **Nerve Growth Factor (NGF)**. In arthritic joints, NGF is overproduced, leading to a state of constant, heightened pain sensitivity. These new injectable drugs work by binding to and neutralizing this excess NGF. By blocking NGF's action, these injections can dramatically reduce arthritis pain for a full month, often with a much wider margin of safety than daily oral NSAIDs because they don't have the same systemic effects on the kidneys or GI tract.

This cutting-edge approach in your pets teaches us a vital lesson for human medicine. It is a perfect model of the "Function Over Numbers" philosophy. The goal is not to eliminate pain at any cost, but to improve function and quality of life with targeted, safer interventions. The existence of these therapies encourages us to be more demanding and creative consumers of human healthcare on Barbara's behalf. It prompts us to ask her doctor:

"Are there any newer, non-opioid options for Mom's arthritis that are more targeted?"

"What about topical NSAID gels or patches that work locally on her knee instead of affecting her whole system?"

"Are there joint injections, like hyaluronic acid or even certain steroids, that could give her a few months of better function?"

Sirius, in his limping grace and his positive response to modern, targeted medicine, guides us toward a more sophisticated and safer model of pain relief for everyone in our house.

Conclusion: The Pawsitive Prescription is for You

In the end, the most profound lessons our pets teach us are often about our own well-being. Leo, with his quiet needs, trains our minds to be better, more observant clinicians for our parents. Sirius, with his boundless affection, directly ministers to our stressed-out souls. The medical system is cold, linear, and transactional. It drains you. Sirius is warm, circular, and unconditional. He restores you. You need the Pawsitive Prescription not just to feel good, but to refuel your tank so you can go back and be the Conductor tomorrow.

Caring for an aging pet is a rehearsal, in many ways, for the journey of human care partnerships. It unfolds on a compressed timeline, teaching us in just a few years what it might take us decades to learn with our human family. It teaches us about the importance of routine, about the wisdom of environmental modification, about patience, about observing subtle signs of pain, and about the bittersweet grace of a life entering its final, poignant chapters.

But most of all, the Pawsitive Prescription is a daily reminder that you, the care partner, need care too. It is a prescription to step away from the overwhelming complexity of human illness and engage in a simple act of uncomplicated love. It is a prescription to take the dog for a walk, not just for his benefit, but for yours—to feel the sun on your face, to move your body, and to connect with a living being whose only request is that you be present. This daily dose of simple, Pawsitive connection is what will give you the strength to continue your vital work. It is the core of the "More Paws" philosophy, the balance to the "Fewer Pills" mission.

CONCLUSION

The Well-Managed House

Do you remember where we began this journey?

You were standing in your mother's kitchen. On the counter sat a chaotic collection of pill bottles, a jumble of prescriptions and supplements that feels confusing, dangerous, and completely out of your control. In that moment, you felt the full, crushing weight of your role: the fear, the exhaustion, the love, and the profound sense of being unprepared for the task ahead.

Now with Fewer Pills, More Paws, the scene is different. The chaos is gone. In its place is a clean, organized **Master Medication List**. Next to it is your **"Go-Bag,"** packed and ready for the hospital, armored with the legal documents that give you a voice. On the fridge is the schedule for your **"Pop-In" visits** to the facility, ensuring Barbara is safe even when you aren't there.

You have not completely fixed the American healthcare system. The fast-paced clinics are still rushing, the pharmacies are still managing incredibly high volumes, and hospitals are still focused on rapid stabilization. But those chaotic forces stop at your front door.

You have built a fortress of advocacy around Barbara. You know about the 8-minute appointment, so you bring a **One-Page Briefing**. You know that the hospital wants to classify her as "Observation," so you ask for an **Admission**. You know that the nursing home might try to sedate her, so you audit the **MAR**.

You are not feeling anxious. You are calmly preparing a protein-rich smoothie for your mother while she reads in the living room. You are also making one for yourself. You finished your own twenty-minute resistance-band workout this morning and slept a solid seven hours last night for the first time in months. After you finish the smoothies, you know you will clip the leash on your good old dog, Sirius, and take him for a brisk, head-clearing walk in the afternoon sun—a non-negotiable part of your day.

Your home is no longer a stressful theater of medical uncertainty. It has become a well-managed house.

This transformation—from chaos to calm, from anxiety to confidence—did not happen by magic. It is the direct result of the knowledge you have gained and the simple, powerful systems you have put in place. It is the result of a fundamental shift in your perspective. You are no longer an accidental caregiver, buffeted by the whims of a confusing healthcare system. You are their care partner. The machine works fast and efficiently. You work for love. And armed with this toolkit, you are the calm, confident conductor of your family's health.

WHAT COMES NEXT?
A TEASER: *THE UNFILTERED BRAIN*

How the Healthcare System Profits from Your Parent's Confusion — and the More Paws Guide to Fighting Back

Author's Note

You've finished *Fewer Pills, More Paws*. You understand homeostenosis. You can see the prescribing cascade. You've learned to observe like Leo.

You are doing everything right.

And yet, it still feels like you're fighting an uphill battle.

Fewer Pills, More Paws taught you important tools. But it's not enough. Understanding your parent's biology is only half the battle.

The other half is understanding why the system is fighting against you—not out of malice, but out of the relentless logic of extraction.

The Unfiltered Brain explains that logic. More importantly, it shows you how to fight it.

Fewer Pills, More Paws made you a Conductor.

The Unfiltered Brain will make you an Advocate.

Prologue: Tuesday to Thursday

Barbara is seventy-eight. Sharp. Independent. She manages

her rose garden and her own taxes.

On Tuesday, she falls and fractures her hip. The surgery is routine; do it all the time, they say. When you visit her post-operative recovery room, she's drowsy but sharp—herself. "Did you water the roses?" she asks, gripping your hand.

You go home confident. You know what to watch for.

By Wednesday evening, she's asking the same question twice. By Thursday morning, she doesn't recognize you. She is pulling at her IV lines and talking to someone that isn't there.

A nurse checks on her, gives her a medication. Barbara becomes sedated. Quiet. Still.

You stand in the hallway trying to understand what happened. It was so fast. So quick.

So automatic.

The charge nurse, very nice, explains: "Severe delirium. The medication will keep her comfortable."

But you have a question no one answers: *How did she go from sharp on Tuesday to this on Thursday?*

What Actually Happened

Barbara's delirium wasn't inevitable. It was constructed, piece by piece, by a system optimized for efficiency at the cost of safety.

Tuesday night: A hospitalist prescribes Trazodone for sleep. He spends four minutes reviewing her chart. The insurance reimbursement system pays him the same whether he spends four minutes or forty. Speed is profitable. Careful prescribing is not.

A pharmacist is covering twice the number of floors that night due to staffing shortages. She doesn't have time to notice the medication interaction or calculate the anticholinergic burden.

Wednesday evening: Barbara develops a fever—a sign of developing infection. A nurse documents it. But she has twelve patients. The time required for observation—to notice that the fever correlates with behavioral change, to catch the infection early—staffing was extracted for cost savings.

The infection goes unnoticed.

Thursday morning: The unit's 24-hour lights have destroyed her circadian rhythm. Her hearing aids are in a drawer at home—never documented on intake because the system's forms capture billing information, not functional needs. She's confused, frightened, isolated in sensory deprivation.

By 9 a.m., she's sedated.

But Here's What Matters

This didn't have to happen.

In hospitals that implement evidence-based protocols designed to prevent delirium, Barbara's story is different. A pharmacist has the time to flag the medication interaction because of a minimum safe staffing law. A nurse, given back the time to spend with patients, she observes the fever and infection early. Protocols calling for darkness at night protects her sleep. Her hearing aids are documented and used.

The delirium might still come. Post-operative vulnerability is real. But it likely would have been milder, and it doesn't escalate to sedation. It resolves with reorientation, with the infection treated, with sleep restored.

These interventions already exist. The research is peer-reviewed. The protocols work. The system fights them not because they don't work, but because they require time, coordination, and a refusal to extract value at the cost of safety. The bottom line is that it affects their bottom line.

Why the System Works Against You

Over the last few decades, value has been systematically extracted from every corner of healthcare. It's the invisible hand of extraction.

Insurance companies deny care to increase profit margins. Private equity firms cut nursing staff to increase returns to investors. Pharmacists cover three floors alone instead of one because of staffing cuts. The billing system pays doctors for speed, not accuracy.

This is not malice. This is efficiency.

But efficiency optimized for profit extraction requires reducing what costs money: time, observation, staffing, coordination, safety.

You cannot extract value without reducing care. You cannot reduce care without making the system less safe.

The uphill battle you feel is real. It's documented. And older adults—just like your parent—are being harmed every day by the system they trust.

The Unfiltered Brain will show you exactly how this extraction happens—with peer-reviewed research naming who profited and how.

But more importantly, it will give you the tools to protect your parent and to refuse to accept the system's extraction as inevitable. Tools that work *now*, in the broken system as it exists.

Leo and Sirius Show Us the Way

The professors return to teach you what a safe system actually looks like.

Sirius shows you the Den Principle: A space designed for recovery has darkness at night, minimal unnecessary noise, familiar presences, careful observation. Not complicated. Not expensive. Just prioritizing patient recovery over system convenience.

Leo teaches the Slow Blink: safety requires time, presence, careful watching. Returning what has been extracted.

When you understand what Leo and Sirius are showing you, you understand what you're fighting for.

What Comes Next

Pick up *The Unfiltered Brain: How the Healthcare System Profits from Your Parent's Confusion — and the More Paws Guide to Fighting Back*

You're not fighting your parent's aging brain. You're fighting a system that extracted safety for profit.

Once you understand that, everything changes.

You become an Advocate.

APPENDIX

The Conductor's Toolkit Templates and Checklists

You have read the science. You have learned the strategy. Now, it is time to do the work.

The following pages contain the specific templates and worksheets referenced throughout the book. They are designed to be your guides to the health care system—transforming vague worries into concrete actionable plans and data to be acted upon.

How to use this section: These forms are not precious. They are tools.

- **Download them**: Find these useful resources at our website **MyRxPro.com**
- **Copy them:** Photocopy these pages or print them out from the digital version of this book.
- **Write on them:** Use a pen. Scribble notes in the margins.
- **Share them:** Hand the *One-Page Briefing* to the doctor. Tape the *Safety Checklist* to the fridge for your siblings to see.

The Tools:
- **Appendix 1: The Master Medication List Template**
  - *The "Brown Bag" audit tool to identify risks and redundancies.*
- **Appendix 2: The One-Page Briefing Template**
  - *The 8-minute appointment planner to ensure your top priorities are heard.*
  - *Estimated Prep Time: 15-30 minutes.*
  - *Estimated Time Saved in Follow-up Calls: 2 Hours*
- **Appendix 3: The Teach-Back Template**
  - *The script to guarantee you understand the doctor's orders before you leave.*
- **Appendix 4: The "Is It Time?" Safety Assessment**
  - *The objective checklist to make data-driven decisions about housing and care.*
- **Appendix 5: The Safety & Driving Observation Log**
  - *The evidence-gathering tool for difficult conversations about independence.*
- **Appendix 6: The "Go-Bag" Checklist**
  - *What to pack in a tote bag to be placed by the door if it's ever time to go to the hospital.*
  - *Prep Time: 30 minutes*
  - *Prevents the #1 cause of hospital medication errors.*
- **Appendix 7: The Dementia (Glacier) vs Delirium (Avalanche) Triage Chart**
  - *Delirium is acute brain failure; this information could save a life.*
- **Appendix 8: The Safe Home Audit: Creating a Safe**

Environment for the Full House
- o *As all members of the household age, creating a safer environment supports function and dignity later in life.*
- *Appendix 9: The Transition Day Checklist*
  - o *A checklist for the first day in the care home.*

The difference between a frantic care partner and a calm Conductor is usually a piece of paper. I hope the following pages and the work you are ready to do will bring you confidence and peace of mind.

Appendix 1: The Master Medication List Template

Download additional copies from MyRxPro.com/caregivers-toolkit

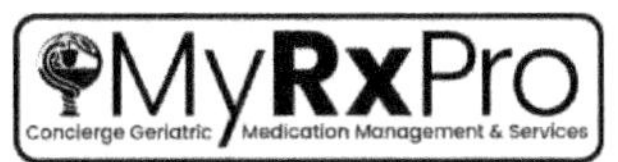

Medication List Template

Patient Name: _______________________________________

Date Updated: ____________________

Allergies: ____

Instructions: The "Brown Bag" Protocol

1. **Gather:** Collect *everything*—prescription bottles, OTCs (Tylenol, Advil), vitamins, supplements, eye drops, and creams.
2. **Transcribe:** Fill out the table below using the information *exactly* as it appears on the bottle.
    1. **Medication Name:** Write down exactly what is on the bottle. Crucially, include both the Brand and Generic names (e.g., Lipitor / Atorvastatin). This prevents the most medical common error: confusing two names for the same drug.
    2. **Dose & Form:** Is it a 10mg tablet? A 50mcg patch? Precision is essential here. A small change in numbers can mean a massive change in effect.
    3. **Instructions:** Copy the instructions exactly. "Take one tablet by mouth twice daily with meals." Those details—with meals, at bedtime—are the rhythm of the drug.
    4. **Prescriber:** Who ordered this? Was it Dr. Evans (Primary) or Dr. Jones (Urology)? You need to know who is directing this particular instrument so you know who to call when there is a problem.
    5. **The "Why" Rule:** If you cannot fill in Column 5 ("What is this for?"), circle that medication. That is your first question for the doctor.

Part 1: The Medication List

1. Medication Name	2. Dose	3. Instructions	4. Prescriber	5. What is this for?
(Brand & Generic)	(e.g., 10mg)	(How and When?)	(Who ordered it?)	(The "Why")
Example: Glucophage/ Metformin	1000 mg	Take 1 with Breakfast and Dinner	Dr Jack Frost	Diabetes

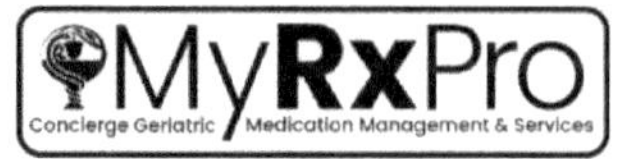

Medication List Template

Part 1: The Medication List (Continued from previous page)

1. Medication Name	2. Dose	3. Instructions	4. Prescriber	5. What is this for?

PART 2: The Pharmacist's Triage (Red Flag Check)

Review your completed list above. Look for these "Red Flags" described in Chapter 7.

- ○ **Duplication:** Is she taking two drugs for the same thing? (e.g., Aleve AND Ibuprofen?) .
- ○ **The Cascade:** Is she taking a drug to fix the side effect of another drug? (e.g., Taking a bladder pill because a water pill makes her pee?) .
- ○ **Beers List Risks:** Is she taking "PM" sleep aids (Benadryl/Diphenhydramine) or Benzodiazepines (Xanax/Ativan)?
- ○ **"As Needed" Rules:** Do you know the maximum number of pain pills she can take in a day? If not, check this box.

Questions for the Pharmacist/Doctor:

____

____

____

____

____

Download additional copies from MyRxPro.com/caregivers-toolkit

Appendix 2: The One-Page Briefing Template

Download additional copies from MyRxPro.com/caregivers-toolkit

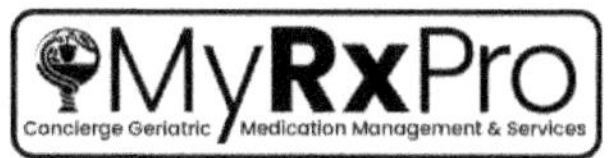

The One-Page Briefing Template

This **One-Page Briefing** template to be used before every doctor's appointment to ensure the 8-minute visit is efficient and productive. Hand this **One-Page Briefing** to the doctor immediately upon entering the room. *"I've put together a one-page summary with our main goals and an updated medication list on the back."*

Patient Name: _______________________________________

Appointment Date: ___________________________________

Physician: ____

I. The "Top 3" Priorities

Do not walk in with a laundry list. Triage your concerns down to the three most urgent issues. If it's not on this list, it waits for next time.

1. **Priority #1:** ___________________________________
   - ○ *Example: "Discuss dizziness since starting amlodipine."*
2. **Priority #2:** ___________________________________
   - ○ *Example: "Explore safer options for arthritis pain."*
3. **Priority #3:** ___________________________________
   - ○ *Example: "Request referral for hearing test."*

II. The Data (Not Drama)

For each priority above, list specific, observable facts. Avoid vague statements like "She seems dizzy." Use dates, times, and specific incidents.

- **Observation Log for Priority #1:**
  - ○ *When:* _______________________________________
  - ○ *What happened:* ____
  - ○ *Frequency:* _________________________________
  - ○ *Triggers (e.g., after morning pills):* _____________________________
- **Observation Log for Priority #2:**
  - ○ *Details:* ____

III. The Attachments

Have these important documents ready in case they are needed

- ○ **Updated Master Medication List** (Includes ALL pills, vitamins, OTCs).
- ○ **Recent Blood Pressure/Blood Sugar Logs** (if applicable).
- ○ **Any other relevant charts, logs, or journals** (e.g., weight, symptoms)

Appendix 3: The Teach-Back Template

Download additional copies from MyRxPro.com/caregivers-toolkit

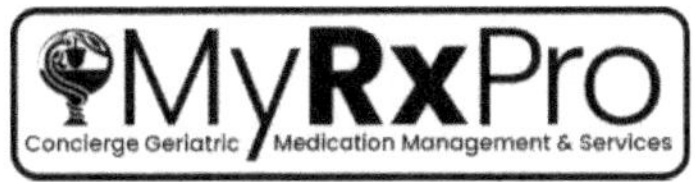

The Teach-Back Template

Use this template script at the end of the appointment to ensure you understand the new plan.

"Let me repeat the plan back to you..."

Medication Changes: ____
Example: "Cut amlodipine to 2.5mg starting tomorrow. Stop Lisinopril."

____

New To-Dos: ____
Example: "Monitor BP twice a week. Call office in 2 weeks."

____

Next Appointment: ____
Example: "Make another appointment in 6 weeks."

____

Other concerns discussed: _______________________________________
Example: "Call about the lab work next week."

____

"Is there anything that I missed?"

____

____

____

____

Appendix 4: The "Is It Time?" Safety Assessment

Download additional copies from MyRxPro.com/caregivers-toolkit

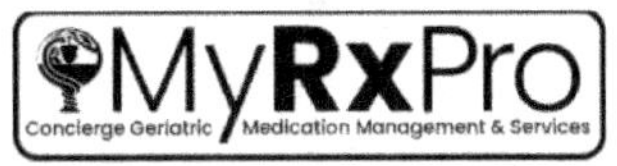

The "Is It Time?" Safety Assessment

This tool is designed to help you make an objective, data-driven assessment of whether "aging in place" is still the safest option for your parent—and for you. Go through this list with a pen and paper. Be brutally honest. There are no right or wrong answers, only clarity. Part 2 of this assessment is just as important.

Part 1: Assessing Your Parent's Needs and Safety
Focus on the reality of the last 6 months.

Falls: Has your parent fallen more than once in the last six months? Are you in a constant state of anxiety about them falling when you are not there? Do they have bruises they can't explain?

○ **Wandering & Safety:** Has your parent ever wandered out of the house and gotten lost? Have you found a stovetop burner left on or the front door left unlocked and open?

○ **Activities of Daily Living (ADLs):** Is your parent consistently unable to perform **two or more** of these core tasks without hands-on help?
- ○ *Bathing*
- ○ *Dressing*
- ○ *Grooming*
- ○ *Eating*
- ○ *Toileting*
- ○ *Transferring (moving from bed to chair)*

○ **Medical Complexity:** Is their medication schedule so complex that you are terrified of making a mistake? Do they require skilled care (injections, wound care, oxygen) you are not trained to provide?

○ **Behavioral Challenges:** If they have dementia, are symptoms like aggression, paranoia, or severe sundowning becoming more than you can safely manage? Are they a danger to themselves or you?

○ **Social Isolation:** Is your parent spending most of their day alone with little interaction beyond your visits? Have they lost connection with friends because it is too difficult to participate?

○ **Home Environment:** Is the house itself unsafe? (e.g., Multi-story with stairs, bathroom too small for a walker, significant clutter/trip hazards).

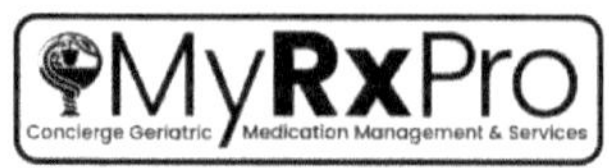

The "Is It Time?" Safety Assessment

This tool is designed to help you make an objective, data-driven assessment of whether "aging in place" is still the safest option for your parent—and for you. Go through this list with a pen and paper. Be brutally honest. There are no right or wrong answers, only clarity. Compare to Part 1.

Part 2: Assessing Your Own Well-Being
You cannot pour from an empty cup. These questions are just as important as Part 1.

○ **Your Physical Health:** Are you chronically sleep-deprived? Have you ignored your own medical appointments? Has lifting or moving your parent caused you physical injury?

○ **Your Mental Health:** Do you feel constant dread, anxiety, or resentment? are you showing signs of depression or loss of interest in things that used to bring you joy?

○ **Your "Why":** Are you providing care at home primarily out of guilt, fear of judgment, or a promise made years ago before you understood the reality?

○ **Your Support System:** Are you the sole care partner with little to no regular help? Do you feel completely alone in this responsibility?

○ **Your Other Responsibilities:** Is your career suffering? Are your relationships with your spouse or children straining to the breaking point?

Interpreting Your Results
If you checked **multiple boxes**—particularly in both sections—it is a clear, data-driven signal that the situation is no longer sustainable. This is not drama; this is not failure. It is an honest compassionate, assessment of safety. A move to a care community is not an act of abandonment. It is the brave, responsible act of admitting that the best possible care (safety, 24/7 supervision, social engagement) is no longer something you can provide alone.

Download additional copies from MyRxPro.com/caregivers-toolkit

Appendix 5: The Safety & Driving Observation Log

Download additional copies from MyRxPro.com/caregivers-toolkit

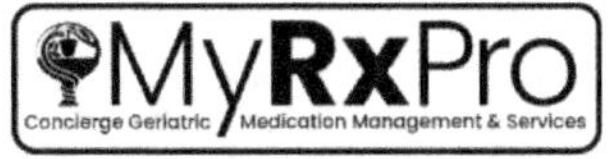

The Safety & Driving Observation Log

Use this log to track specific, objective events over a 2-week period. Be a "silent observer" like your cat, Leo. Do not critique in the moment; simply record the data. This document is your evidence for the doctor.

Part 1: The Driving Log

Ride as a passenger. Watch for: **Close Calls** *(braking/swerving),* **Vehicle Control** *(drifting/abrupt braking/slow speed)* **Cognitive Gaps** *(getting lost/missed a traffic sign/delayed reaction)*

Date & Time	Event Type (Check One)	Description of Incident (Be Specific)
Ex: 10/14, 2pm	○ Close Call ○ Confusion ○ Control	*Drifted into left lane on Main St; oncoming car honked.*
	○ Close Call ○ Confusion ○ Control	
	○ Close Call ○ Confusion ○ Control	
	○ Close Call ○ Confusion ○ Control	

Physical Evidence Check:

○ Unexplained fresh scrapes or dents on the vehicle? (Date noted: ___________)
○ Curb damage to tires or rims?
○ Other damage, be specific___________________

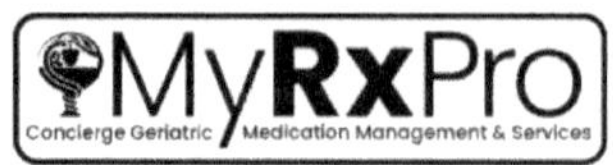

The Safety & Driving Observation Log

Use this log to track specific, objective events over a 2-week period. Be a "silent observer" like your cat, Leo. Do not critique in the moment; simply record the data. This document is your evidence for the doctor.

Part 2: Home Safety Log
*The same cognitive gaps that affect driving often show up at home first. Look for: **Burnt pans, unlocked doors, "furniture walking" (using furniture for balance), medical attention for injuries, falls, or unexplained bruises***

Date & Time	Observation	Why it concerns you
Ex: 11/2, 10pm	*Stove burner left on High.*	*Fire risk; Did not know who turned it on.*

Download additional copies from MyRxPro.com/caregivers-toolkit

Appendix 6: The "Go-Bag" Checklist

Download additional copies from MyRxPro.com/caregivers-toolkit

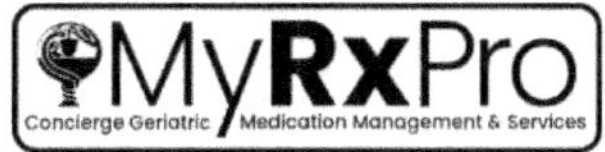

The Hospital "Go-Bag" Checklist

Instructions: Photocopy this page, or download a copy from MyRxPro.com. Pack the items listed below into a brightly colored tote bag and keep it by your front door. When the ambulance is called, you do not have time to think. Grab this bag.

☑ **The Critical Documents**

These are your "Ticket to Entry" and your "Shield."

○ **Master Medication List:** Two copies (one for the ER doctor, one for the nurse). *Tip: Put all current pill bottles into a Ziploc bag and throw them in, too.*

○ **Medical Power of Attorney (MPOA):** A photocopy of your Medical POA. (Sometimes called a HCPOA)

○ **Financial Power of Attorney / Durable Power of Attorney:** A photocopy of your Financial POA. (Sometimes just called the POA)

○ **Living will / POLST Form:** Living will are resuscitation wishes of your parent. POLST is the pink or green form are physician order dictating resuscitation orders.

○ **ID & Insurance Cards:** Photocopies of the front and back of her insurance/Medicare cards and photo ID.

☑ **The Sensory Kit**

Hospitals are sensory deprivation chambers. Protect her input channels to prevent delirium.

○ **Hearing Aids:** Plus extra batteries and the charger.

○ **Glasses:** In a hard case labeled with her name.

○ **Dentures:** Plus a labeled denture cup and adhesive.

☑ **Comfort & Anchors**

Humanize them to the staff and soothe her amygdala.

○ **One Familiar Item:** A small fleece blanket or a shawl that reminds them of home.

○ **One Family Photo:** Tape this to the wall or bed rail. It gives your loved one an anchor to who they are and It reminds busy staff that this patient is a person who is loved.

○ **Phone Charger:** For *your* phone. It's going to be a long night.

☑ **The "STOP" Sign**

Write the following on a bright Neon Index Card and tape it to the top of the Medication List.

ATTENTION: SENSITIVE BRAIN Patient has a history of Cognitive Decline.

1. **NO Benadryl (Diphenhydramine)**
2. **NO Benzodiazepines (Ativan/Xanax)** *These medications cause immediate Delirium/Agitation for this patient.*

If Agitated: Please call family/POA first to assist with calming.

Appendix

Appendix 7: The Dementia (Glacier) vs Delirium (Avalanche) Triage Chart

Download additional copies from MyRxPro.com/caregivers-toolkit

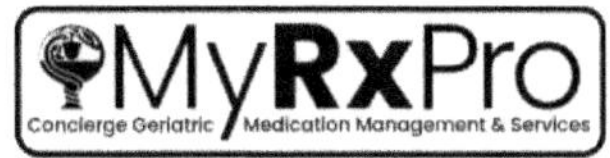

The Dementia (Glacier) vs. Delirium (Avalanche) Triage Chart

Instructions: If your parent is acting "strange," stop. Do not assume it is just "dementia getting worse." Use this chart to check for Delirium.

The Sign	Dementia (The Glacier)	Delirium (The Avalanche)
Speed of Onset	**Slow.** Changes happen over months or years. You look back and realize they are worse than last Christmas.	**Sudden.** Changes happen over hours or days. They were fine at breakfast but confused by dinner.
Attention	**Generally Alert.** They may forget *what* you said, but they are looking at you and paying attention.	**Zoning Out.** They cannot focus. They drift off mid-sentence, look glassy-eyed, or seem "out of it."
Sleep	**Fragmented.** They might wake up at night, but they have a general routine.	**Disturbed.** They are lethargic and un-wakeable during the day, or hyper-alert and up all night.
Speech	**Word-Finding.** "Pass me the... thing." They struggle to find the right noun.	**Incoherent.** They are slurring words, speaking gibberish, or talking to people who aren't there.
The Cause	**Brain Atrophy.** A progressive structural change.	**A Medical Crisis.** Infection (UTI), Dehydration, Medication Toxicity, or Pain is causing this.
YOUR ACTION	**Use the Paws Protocol.** Use Tone, Touch, and Tempo to soothe.	**MEDICAL EMERGENCY.** This is brain failure. Call the doctor or go to the ER immediately.

Appendix 8: The Safe Home Audit: Creating a Safe Environment for the Full House

Download additional copies from MyRxPro.com/caregivers-toolkit

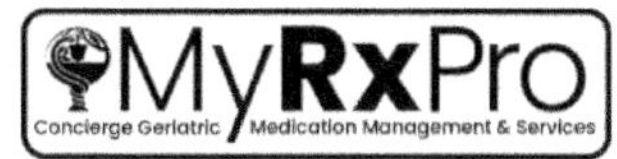

The Safe Home Audit

Creating a Safe Environment for the Full House

Instructions: Walk through your home with "Fresh Eyes." We are looking for areas where physics works against the safety of an older adult. Research as shown these are the dangers to look out for.

☑ **The Floors (The Terrain)**

○ **Remove ALL Throw Rugs:**

- o These are the #1 trip hazard for walkers and shuffling gaits. A catch of the toe can lead to a hip fracture.
- o *Bonus:* Removing them also helps old dogs who slip on shifting fabrics.

○ **Secure Cords:** Tape down lamp cords running across walkways.

- o Prevents entanglement and tripping.

☑ **The Lighting (The Horizon)**

○ **Motion-Sensor Nightlights:** Install in the hallway, bathroom, and bedroom.

- o Prevents falls during late-night bathroom trips by providing visual cues for balance.
- o *Bonus:* Helps pets with failing vision navigate without bumping into walls.

○ **Reduce Glare:** Close blinds at sunset.

- o Prevents "Sundowning" shadows that trigger confusion and visual hallucinations.

☑ **The Stairs (The High Risk Zone)**

○ **Contrast Tape:** Place a strip of bright/neon tape on the edge of every step.

- o Older eyes lose depth perception. The tape clearly defines where the step ends so she doesn't miss a riser.
- o *Bonus:* Helps pets see the drop-off.

○ **Double Handrails:** Ensure there are rails on *both* sides of the stairwell so they can use both arms for leverage.

☑ **The Furniture (The Flow)**

○ **Create Wide "Runways":** Can you walk through the living room with a walker without turning sideways? If not, move the coffee table.

○ **Stable Seating:** Ensure their favorite chair has firm arms. She needs to be able to push herself up using her triceps, not just her legs.

Appendix 9: The Transition Day Checklist.

Download additional copies from MyRxPro.com/caregivers-toolkit

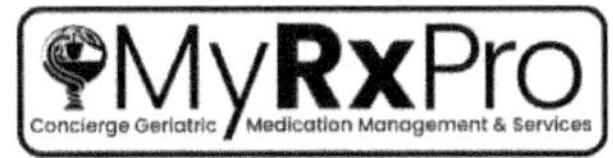

The Transition Day Checklist

When to use this: On the day your loved one moves into a Skilled Nursing Facility (SNF), Rehab Center, or Assisted Living Facility.
Goal: To transfer critical information ("The Baton") effectively and ensure the physical environment is safe before you leave the building.

Part 1: The "Face Sheet" (Bring 3 Copies)
Do not rely on the hospital to send the records. Systems fail. You are the courier. Create a single-page document with the following information in large, bold type. Hand one copy to the **Director of Nursing**, one to the **Unit Manager**, and tape one to the **wall inside the room** (if allowed).
- **Patient Name & Preferred Name:** (e.g., "Barbara Smith, prefers 'Barb'")
- **Primary Contact:** Your Name & Cell Phone Number.
- **Code Status:** (DNR / DNI / Full Code) — *Attach a copy of the POLST/MOLST form.*
- **The "Big Three" Alerts:**
  - ○ Fall Risk (e.g., "Tries to get up without help at night")
  - ○ Swallowing/Choking Risk (e.g., "Needs thickened liquids")
  - ○ Allergies (e.g., "Penicillin," "Latex")
- **Current Medication List:** A clean list of what she is actually taking.
- **Baseline Status:** A one-sentence description of her "Normal." (e.g., *"Barb is usually confused in the mornings but clear in the evenings. She can feed herself but needs help cutting meat."*)

Part 2: The Room Sweep (Safety Check)
Perform this check immediately upon entering the room. Do not unpack until these are verified.
The Bed:
- ○ Is the bed at the lowest possible height setting?
- ○ Are the brakes locked on the bed wheels?
- ○ Is the mattress firm/stable?

The Path:
- ○ Is the path from the bed to the bathroom clear of cords, rugs, or furniture?
- ○ Is the floor dry and non-slip?

The Equipment:
- ○ **Call Light:** Is it plugged in? Does it work? Is it clipped within reach of the pillow?
- ○ **Assist Bars:** Are the grab bars in the bathroom secure (give them a hard shake)?
- ○ **Oxygen/Suction:** (If applicable) Are the lines connected and flowing?

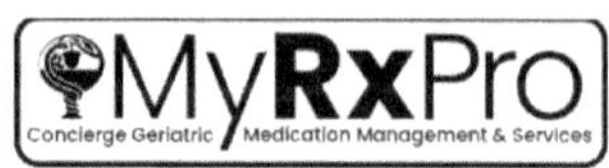

Part 3: The Staff Handoff (The "Conductor" Meeting)
Do not leave the facility until you have made eye contact with these specific people. Do not settle for the front desk receptionist.
Identify the Unit Manager:
- ○ Ask: *"Who is the nurse in charge of this specific hallway/unit?"*
- ○ Action: Introduce yourself. *"I am [Name]. I want to be a partner, not a pest. If I see a safety issue, are you the right person to call?"*
- ○ **Get the Number:** Ask for the direct line to the Nurses' Station (not the main lobby number).

Identify the CNA (Certified Nursing Assistant):
- • *This is the person who will actually touch/move your parent.*
- ○ Action: Share one "Human Fact" to build connection. (e.g., *"She loves dogs," "She used to be a teacher."*)
- ○ Action: Share the "Trigger." (e.g., *"If she says she wants to go home, she usually just needs to use the restroom."*)

Part 4: The "Paws" (Comfort Anchors)
The goal is to reduce cortisol (stress) to prevent delirium.
- ○ **Scent/Touch:** A familiar pillow with a bright, recognizable pillowcase.
- ○ **Visual:** A large photo of family or pets placed where she can see it from the bed.
- ○ **Auditory:** Noise-canceling headphones or a white noise machine if the hallway is loud.
- ○ **The "Go-Bag" Transfer:** Ensure her glasses, hearing aids (with batteries), and dentures are in the room and labeled with her name.

Part 5: The Exit Protocol
- ○ Confirm the staff knows you are leaving.
- ○ Ensure the Call Light is in your parent's hand.
- ○ Say goodbye. (Keep it brief to minimize agitation).
- ○ **Go home and sleep.**

Download additional copies from MyRxPro.com/caregivers-toolkit

REFERENCES

Introduction
1. Aronson L. Elderhood: Redefining Aging, Transforming Medicine, Reimagining Life. New York, NY: Bloomsbury Publishing; 2019.

Chapter 1: The 55-Year-Old at the Crossroads
1. Aronson L. Elderhood: Redefining Aging, Transforming Medicine, Reimagining Life. New York, NY: Bloomsbury Publishing; 2019.
2. Lakatta EG, Levy D. Arterial and cardiac aging: major shareholders in cardiovascular disease enterprises: Part I: aging arteries: a "set up" for vascular disease. Circulation. 2003;107(1):139-146.
3. Rosenberg IH. Sarcopenia: origins and clinical relevance. J Nutr. 1997;127(5):990S-991S.
4. Cruz-Jentoft AJ, Baeyens JP, Bauer JM, et al. Sarcopenia: European consensus on definition and diagnosis: Report of the European Working Group on Sarcopenia in Older People. Age Ageing. 2010;39(4):412-423.
5. DeFronzo RA. The Triumvirate: β-Cell, Muscle, Liver. A Collusion Responsible for NIDDM. Diabetes. 1981;30(9):1000-1004.
6. Weinstein JR, Anderson S. The aging kidney: physiological changes. Adv Chronic Kidney Dis. 2010;17(4):302-307.
7. Sapolsky RM. Glucocorticoids and hippocampal atrophy in neuropsychiatric disorders. Arch Gen Psychiatry. 2000;57(10):925-935.
8. Xie L, Kang H, Xu Q, et al. Sleep drives metabolite clearance from the adult brain. Science. 2013;342(6156):373-377.

Chapter 2: The Stradivarius
1. Aronson L. Elderhood: Redefining Aging, Transforming Medicine, Reimagining Life. New York, NY: Bloomsbury Publishing; 2019.
2. Fries JF. Aging, natural death, and the compression of morbidity. N Engl J Med. 1980;303(3):130-135.
3. Lakatta EG, Ferrucci L. The Fulfilling Symphony of Heart and Vessels Interacting in the Tune of Life and Successful Aging. Circulation.

2003;108(16):1909-1913.

4. Fliser D, Franek E, Ritz E. Renal function in the elderly—is it a matter of age or disease? Nephrol Dial Transplant. 1997;12(10):2038-2040.

5. Schmucker DL. Liver function and aging: a historical perspective. In: Liver and Aging. Humana Press; 2001:3-10.

6. Morley JE, Baumgartner RN, Roubenoff R, et al. Sarcopenia. J Lab Clin Med. 2001;137(4):231-243.

7. Fried LP, Tangen CM, Walston J, et al. Frailty in older adults: evidence for a phenotype. J Gerontol A Biol Sci Med Sci. 2001;56(3):M146-M157.

8. Russell RM. Changes in gastrointestinal function attributed to aging. Am J Clin Nutr. 1992;55(6):1203S-1207S.

9. Pawelec G, Larbi A. Immunosenescence and vaccination in the elderly. Neuroimmunomodulation. 2008;15(4-6):241-245.

10. Franceschi C, Bonafe M, Valensin S, et al. Inflamm-aging. An evolutionary perspective on immunosenescence. Ann N Y Acad Sci. 2000;908(1):244-254.

11. Taquet M, Todd JA, Harrison PJ. The recombinant shingles vaccine is associated with lower risk of dementia. Nat Med. 2024;30:1786–1793.

12. Stern Y. What is cognitive reserve? Theory and research application of the reserve concept. J Int Neuropsychol Soc. 2002;8(3):448-460.

13. Farage MA, Miller KW, Elsner P, Maibach HI. Intrinsic and extrinsic factors in skin ageing: a review. Int J Cosmet Sci. 2008;30(2):87-95.

Chapter 3: The Principle of Less is More

1. Bosch G, Hagen-Plantinga EA, Hendriks WH. Dietary nutrient profiles of wild wolves: insights for optimal dog nutrition? Br J Nutr. 2015;113(S1):S40-S54.

2. Court MH. Feline drug metabolism and disposition: pharmacokinetic evidence for shared and unique pathways. J Vet Pharmacol Ther. 2013;36(3):215-225.

3. Tegeder I, Lötsch J. The impact of polymorphisms in the main metabolizing enzymes and transporters of NSAIDs on their analgesic efficacy and gastrointestinal toxicity. Eur J Clin Pharmacol. 2009;65(9):857-863.

4. MacDonald ML, Rogers QR, Morris JG. Nutrition of the domestic cat, a mammalian carnivore. Annu Rev Nutr. 1984;4:521-562.

5. Vandeweerd JM, Coisnon C, Grulke S, et al. Systematic review of efficacy of nutraceuticals to alleviate clinical signs of osteoarthritis. J Vet Intern Med. 2012;26(3):448-456.

6. Salvin HE, McGreevy PD, Sachdev PS, Valenzuela MJ. Under diagnosis of canine cognitive dysfunction: a cross-sectional survey of older companion dogs. Vet J. 2011;188(1):36-41.

Chapter 4: The Coordination Gap

1. Tai-Seale M, McGuire TG, Zhang W. Time allocation in primary care office visits. *Health Aff (Millwood)*. 2007;26(5):1873-1883.
2. Schommer JC, Pedersen CA, Gaither CA, et al. Pharmacists' desired and actual times in work activities: evidence of a gap from the 2004 National Pharmacist Workforce Study. *J Am Pharm Assoc*. 2006;46(3):340-347.
3. Quinn K. After the revolution: DRGs at age 30. *Ann Intern Med*. 2014;160(6):426-429.
4. Lapi F, Azoulay L, Yin H, Nessim SJ, Suissa S. Concurrent use of diuretics, angiotensin converting enzyme inhibitors, and angiotensin receptor blockers with non-steroidal anti-inflammatory drugs and risk of acute kidney injury: nested case-control study. *BMJ*. 2013;346:e8525.

Chapter 5: The Conductor

1. Annas GJ. HIPAA regulations - a new era of medical-record privacy? *N Engl J Med*. 2003;348(15):1486-1490.
2. Bomba PA, Kemp M, Bates JS. POLST: An improvement over traditional advance directives. *Cleve Clin J Med*. 2012;79(7):457-464.
3. Nathan A, Goodyer L, Lovejoy A, Rashid A. 'Brown bag' medication reviews as a means of optimizing patients' use of medication and of identifying potential clinical problems. *Fam Pract*. 1999;16(3):278-282.

Chapter 6: Interrupting the Prescribing Cascade

1. Rochon PA, Gurwitz JH. Optimising drug treatment for elderly people: the prescribing cascade. BMJ. 1997;315(7115):1096-1099.
2. Eriksson T, Gustafson Y, Fagerström L, et al. Drug-related urinary incontinence in the elderly: a cross-sectional study. Drugs Aging. 2016;33(3):221-229.
3. Campbell N, Boustani M, Lane K, et al. The cognitive impact of anticholinergics: a clinical review. Clin Interv Aging. 2019;14:2235–2243.
4. Gray SL, Anderson ML, Dublin S, et al. Cumulative use of strong anticholinergics and incident dementia: a prospective cohort study. JAMA Intern Med. 2015;175(3):401-407.
5. Richardson K, Fox C, Maidment I, et al. Anticholinergic drugs and risk of dementia: case-control study. BMJ. 2018;361:k1315.
6. American Geriatrics Society Beers Criteria® Update Expert Panel. American Geriatrics Society 2023 updated AGS Beers Criteria® for potentially inappropriate medication use in older adults. J Am Geriatr Soc. 2023;71(7):2052-2081.
7. Appel LJ, Moore TJ, Obarzanek E, et al. A clinical trial of the effects of dietary patterns on blood pressure. N Engl J Med. 1997;336(16):1117-1124.

References

8. Neter JE, Stam BE, Kok FJ, et al. Influence of weight reduction on blood pressure: a meta-analysis. Hypertension. 2003;42(5):878-884.

9. Dumoulin C, Cacciari LP, Hay-Smith EJ. Pelvic floor muscle training versus no treatment, or inactive control treatments, for urinary incontinence in women. Cochrane Database Syst Rev. 2018;10(10):CD005654.

10. Szuhany KL, Bugatti M, Otto MW. A meta-analytic review of the effects of exercise on brain-derived neurotrophic factor. J Psychiatr Res. 2015;60:56-64.

11. Northey JM, Cherbuin N, Pumpa KL, et al. Exercise interventions for cognitive function in adults older than 50: a systematic review with meta-analysis. Br J Sports Med. 2018;52(3):154-160.

Chapter 7: The Path to Fewer Pills, More Paws

1. Ngandu T, Lehtisalo J, Solomon A, et al. A 2-year multidomain intervention of diet, exercise, cognitive training, and vascular risk monitoring versus control to prevent cognitive decline in at-risk elderly people (FINGER): a randomised controlled trial. Lancet. 2015;385(9984):2255-2263.

2. Baker LD, Kivipelto M, et al. U.S. POINTER: Study design and baseline characteristics of a 2-year randomized controlled trial to prevent cognitive decline. Alzheimers Dement. 2023;19(11):5256-5267.

3. Solomon A, Turunen H, Ngandu T, et al. Effect of the Apolipoprotein E Genotype on Cognitive Change During a Multidomain Lifestyle Intervention: A Subgroup Analysis of a Randomized Clinical Trial. JAMA Neurol. 2018;75(4):462-470.

4. Kraemer WJ, Ratamess NA. Fundamentals of resistance training: progression and exercise prescription. Med Sci Sports Exerc. 2004;36(4):674-688.

5. Morris MC, Tangney CC, Wang Y, et al. MIND diet associated with reduced incidence of Alzheimer's disease. Alzheimers Dement. 2015;11(9):1007-1014.

6. Bauer J, Biolo G, Cederholm T, et al. Evidence-based recommendations for optimal dietary protein intake in older people: a position paper from the PROT-AGE Study Group. J Am Med Dir Assoc. 2013;14(8):542-559.

7. Valdes AM, Walter J, Segal E, Spector TD. Role of the gut microbiome in nutrition and health. BMJ. 2018;361:k2179.

8. The SPRINT MIND Investigators for the SPRINT Research Group. Effect of Intensive Blood-Pressure Control on Risk of Dementia and Cognitive Impairment. JAMA. 2019;321(6):553-561.

9. Xie L, Kang H, Xu Q, et al. Sleep drives metabolite clearance from the adult brain. Science. 2013;342(6156):373-377.

10. Tähkämö L, Partonen T, Pesonen AK. Systematic review of light exposure impact on human circadian rhythm. Chronobiol Int. 2019;36(2):151-170.

11. Gerritsen RJ, Band GP. Breath of life: the respiratory vagal stimulation model of contemplative activity. Front Hum Neurosci. 2018;12:397.

Chapter 10: Safe At Home

1. Pomidor A, ed. Clinician's Guide to Assessing and Counseling Older Drivers. 4th ed. New York: American Geriatrics Society; 2019.

2. Adler G, Rottunda S. The driver retirement decision: A comparison of self-reported and state-recorded crash and violation data. Gerontologist. 2006;46(3):354-359.

3. O'Neill D. Driving and dementia. J R Soc Med. 2015;108(4):131-135.

4. Bowen M. Family Therapy in Clinical Practice. New York: Jason Aronson; 1978.

5. Chihuri S, Mielenz TJ, DiMaggio CJ, et al. Driving cessation and health outcomes in older adults. J Am Geriatr Soc. 2016;64(2):332-341.

6. The Hartford Center for Mature Market Excellence & MIT AgeLab. At the Crossroads: Family Conversations About Driving. 2010.

Chapter 11: The Unfiltered Brain

1. Tales A, Snowden RJ, Haworth J, Wilcock G. Abnormal visual search in Alzheimer's disease and mild cognitive impairment. *J Sleep Res.* 2002;11(4):303-314.

2. Reisberg B, Franssen EH, Hasan SM, et al. Retrogenesis: clinical, physiologic, and pathologic mechanisms in brain aging, Alzheimer's and other dementing processes. *Eur Arch Psychiatry Clin Neurosci.* 1999;249 Suppl 3:28-36.

3. McKeith IG, Boeve BF, Dickson DW, et al. Diagnosis and management of dementia with Lewy bodies: Fourth consensus report of the DLB Consortium. *Neurology.* 2017;89(1):88-100.

4. Snow T. *The GEMS® Brain Change Model.* Positive Approach to Care. Accessed March 2026. https://teepasnow.com/about/about-teepa-snow/the-gems-brain-change-model/

Chapter 12: The Paws Protocol

1. Rizzolatti G, Craighero L. The mirror-neuron system. *Annu Rev Neurosci.* 2004;27:169-192.

2. Schirmer A, Kotz SA. Beyond the right hemisphere: brain mechanisms mediating vocal emotional processing. *Trends Cogn Sci.* 2006;10(1):24-30.

3. von Muggenthaler E. The felid purr: a healing mechanism? *J Acoust*

   Soc Am. 2001;110(5):2666.
4. Snow T. Understanding the Changing Brain: A Positive Approach to Dementia Care. Positive Approach, LLC; 2022.
5. Salthouse TA. The processing-speed theory of adult age differences in cognition. *Psychol Rev.* 1996;103(3):403-428.

Chapter 13: Delirium, The Avalanche
1. Inouye SK, Westendorp RG, Saczynski JS. Delirium in elderly people. *Lancet.* 2014;383(9920):911-922.
2. Fong TG, Tulebaev SR, Inouye SK. Delirium in elderly adults: diagnosis, prevention and treatment. *Nat Rev Neurol.* 2009;5(4):210-220.
3. Mayne S, Bowden A, Sundvall PD, Gunnarsson R. The scientific evidence for a potential link between confusion and urinary tract infection in the elderly is still confusing - a systematic literature review. *BMC Geriatr.* 2019;19(1):32.
4. Lin FR, Yaffe K, Xia J, et al. Hearing Loss and Cognitive Decline in Older Adults. *JAMA Intern Med.* 2013;173(4):293–299.
5. Husebo BS, Ballard C, Sandvik R, Nilsen OB, Aarsland D. Efficacy of treating pain to reduce behavioural disturbances in residents of nursing homes with dementia: cluster randomised clinical trial. *BMJ.* 2011;343:d4065.

Chapter 17: Lessons in Appetite and Agency from the Finicky Cat
1. Gunn-Moore D, Moffat K, Christie LA, Head E. Cognitive dysfunction and the neurobiology of aging in cats. J Small Anim Pract. 2007;48(10):546-553.
2. Landsberg GM, Araujo JA. Behavior problems in geriatric pets. Vet Clin North Am Small Anim Pract. 2005;35(3):675-698.
3. Clarke SP, Bennett D. Feline osteoarthritis: a prospective study of 28 cases. J Small Anim Pract. 2006;47(8):439-445.

Chapter 18: Lessons in Mobility and Joy from the Good Old Dog
1. Beetz A, Uvnäs-Moberg K, Julius H, Kotrschal K. Psychosocial and psychophysiological effects of human-animal interactions: the possible role of oxytocin. Front Psychol. 2012;3:234.
2. Kraus C, et al. Efficacy and safety of bedinvetmab for the treatment of pain associated with osteoarthritis in dogs. Vet Anaesth Analg. 2021;48(6):925-937.
3. Gruen ME, et al. Long-term safety, efficacy and client-perceived quality of life associated with frunevetmab for the control of pain from osteoarthritis in cats. J Vet Intern Med. 2021;35(4):1832-1843.

Acknowledgments

To Anastasia Gilliam, my constant confidante and support for MyRxPro.com. Thank you for helping me realize my dreams. I couldn't do it without you.

To my mentors at Virginia Commonwealth University, Oregon Health & Science University, and Yale University: thank you for your patience and kindness, for being phenomenal teachers, and the generosity of your time. To Jürgen Venitz, MD, PhD for teaching me how to be a scientist, teacher, and a generous mentor. To Patricia Slattum, PharmD, PhD, for teaching me that the best medicine is often the one we have the courage to stop. To Elizabeth Eckstrom, MD, MPH, for believing in me. To Mary Tinetti, MD, Thomas Gill, MD, and Sean Jeffery, PharmD, BCGP, FASCP, AGSF for instilling in me a rigorous commitment to geriatric science and exceptional patient care.

To the care partners I have had the pleasure of working with over the years. And, to those who subscribe to the newsletter at MyRxPro.com and watch my videos on YouTube: your questions and your challenges are the fuel for this work. This book is for all of you.

To Boris, Natasha, Sophie, Thelonious, Midnight, and Pearl, my other "professors." You are my teachers of wisdom, joy, and comfort.

Finally, my children: thank you for your love and patience. To Monica Franz for your many years of support. To Sam Lee and Amy Senkbiel, my siblings and friends. And to my own parents, who taught me that the best wisdom comes from hard work and compassion.

David Lee, PharmD, PhD is the founder of **MyRxPro.com**, a service and platform dedicated to demystifying the medicine cabinet for family care partners. A former Yale Fellow in Geriatric Clinical Epidemiology, David has spent his career at the intersection of complex science, research, and senior care.

He is the author of *Fewer Pills, More Paws*, a guide born from a simple observation: sometimes less is more. Through his YouTube channel and the *MyRxPro Newsletter*, he has earned a reputation for translating dense medical data into practical, compassionate wisdom.

Beyond his writing, David provides direct support to families navigating the healthcare maze. Through private medication consultations and care partnership coaching, he acts as a care advocate for complex cases, helping families untangle overwhelmed medication lists and find clarity.

David earned his PharmD and PhD from Virginia Commonwealth University. He lives and works in Portland,

Oregon with his two wonderful kids and two finicky cats, Pearl and Midnight.

Connect with David: For video guides, templates, and newsletters:

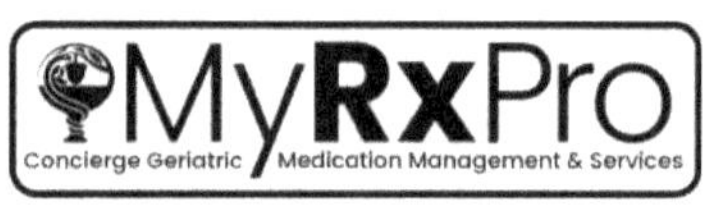

MyRxPro.com